D0859977

an extra pair
of hands

Kate Mosse

an extra pair of hands

A story of caring, ageing & everyday acts of love

PROFILE BOOKS

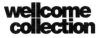

First published in Great Britain in 2021 by
PROFILE BOOKS LTD
29 Cloth Fair
London
EC1A 7JQ
www.profilebooks.co.uk

Published in association with Wellcome Collection

wellcome
collection

183 Euston Road
London NW1 2BE
www.wellcomecollection.org

10 9 8 7 6 5 4 3 2 1

Typeset in Freight Text by MacGuru Ltd
Designed by Barneby Ltd
Printed and bound in Great Britain by Clays Ltd, Elcograf S.p.A.

A CIP record for this book can be obtained from the British Library

ISBN: 978 1 78816 261 6
eISBN: 978 1 78283 551 6
Audio ISBN: 978 1 78283 885 2

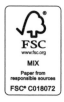

FSC
www.fsc.org
MIX
Paper from
responsible sources
FSC® C018072

As always, for my beloved Greg, Martha and Felix

With love and admiration for my much-missed parents
Richard Hugh Mosse
(30 May 1924 – 18 May 2011)
Barbara Mary Mosse
(15 September 1931 – 21 December 2014)

And for my wonderful mother-in-law
Rosemary Turner – aka Granny Rosie
(2 November 1930 – still going strong!)

Freedom. It isn't once, to walk out
under the Milky Way, feeling the rivers
of light, the fields of dark –
freedom is daily, prose-bound, routine
remembering. Putting together, inch by inch,
the starry worlds. From all the lost collections.

Adrienne Rich

from 'For Memory', 1979

Contents

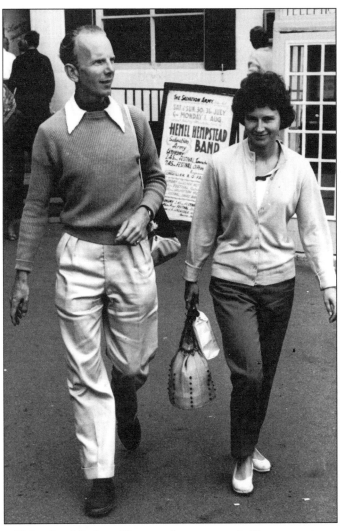

Richard and Barbara Mosse on honeymoon in Guernsey, 1954

Christmas 1975

MY SISTERS AND I are sitting in the back of the car, our legs touching, and the seat scratchy.

Street lights flash by in quiet suburban towns, then we're out into the darkness of country roads in the South Downs. Sleepy after a long day, a visit to my mother's favourite cousin and his wife, somewhere in Surrey. Sandwiches for the journey home. Edam cheese, something I've never eaten before. I want to like it, but it doesn't taste of anything and it's the texture of my swimming hat.

It's winter and we're wearing flared jeans and striped polo necks, itchy at the neck. Beige and mustard yellow, the colours of the 1970s. Lava lamp prints. Or maybe not. Memory is a fickle friend and there were many journeys to relatives at Christmas.

But if the image is slightly blurred, I'm certain it's

Boxing Day or thereabouts, coming up for six o'clock. We're in our usual places – me behind our mother on the passenger side, my middle sister perched and looking straight ahead, my youngest sister curled up behind our father, a folded coat against the window for a pillow. In the compartment beneath the handbrake, there's a packet of tissues and a metal tin of car sweets – Fox's Glacier Mints and barley sugars, the brittle taste of day trips.

I wipe the inside of the glass with my sleeve and ask if the radio can be turned on. The relief! We're just in time for the tail end of the Top 20 and the Christmas No. 1.

In those days before personalised playlists and twenty-four-hour sound, the Radio 1 countdown on a Sunday night was a ritual. One of those things that made girls growing up in villages in Sussex feel connected to something bigger, beyond the realms of our lived experience. For the fifth week running, it's Queen with 'Bohemian Rhapsody'. I've seen the video on *Top of the Pops* and, as I listen, I picture that split screen dividing into boxes, then dividing again and again. Singing along under my breath to words I don't understand, yet relishing the sound of them, the spirit of them, the promise of them.

I am fourteen and young for my age, but wanting to fit in with the more popular pupils at my 2,000-strong girls' comp, the ones who smoke and have boyfriends, who roll their skirts up and wear platform shoes to school.

Blue eyeshadow. Imagine.

I'm not sure why I remember this journey so clearly, when in truth it could have been any other December in the 1970s: perhaps visiting my maternal uncle and aunt in Addlestone (though I think that year the Christmas No. 1 was Slade) or an afternoon spent with my paternal grandparents in Hove. Memories fragment, slip and slide, put themselves back together like a kaleidoscope. Playing 'I Spy' to pass the time until we're bored of it. The ritual of seeing which of us could count the most Christmas trees in the windows of all the houses and flats as we drove along the old coast road from East to West Sussex, until the spire of Chichester Cathedral welcomed us home. Knowing that, because it was the holidays, we'd have supper on our laps in front of the television. Knowing my father would have left the light on in the porch so we didn't come back to a dark house and that our Christmas tree would be sparkling red and blue. A holly wreath on the front door. Knowing all this in advance because this was how it always was.

I didn't, then, realise how exceptional this quiet, ordered childhood was, how ordinary and how precious. Knowing that I was loved. And because of those very many years of being loved unconditionally, and supported unconditionally, that what was required some thirty-five years later would be both possible and a privilege.

This is not a 'how to' book for the 8.8 million adults in the UK who find themselves carers, nor a social analysis of the structures and inequalities in the UK care system. Though there are common challenges, everyone's experience is unique. My husband, our children, my sisters, my brother-in-law would write different stories of these same times and their roles as carers.

Rather, it's a tribute to three extraordinary people – my father, my mother and my mother-in-law – and my own personal reflections about what it means to find oneself, in middle age, as an 'extra pair of hands'. It's about the nature of memory, about celebrating older people and ageing, about gentle heroism, about invisibility, about family and history, about complexity, about trying and failing simultaneously, about the juggling of work deadlines, about unreliability, about exhaustion and never getting a full night's sleep, about the numbing repetition of everyday tasks, about grief, about patience, compassion and empathy, guilt and loss, about the right to die with dignity, about reciprocity, about our brilliant NHS, about learning to embrace a different pace of life, about our fading selves, about regret, about absence, about partnership, about liberation, about being lucky enough to be in a position to repay a lifetime of caring.

But most of all, it's a story about love.

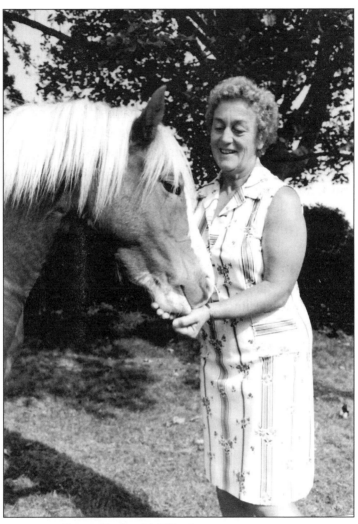

Granny Rosie with Filly, Sussex, summer 1974

1

Three Generations

IT STARTED with Granny Rosie.

When my husband and I left London in 1998, and came home to Sussex with our two young children, we asked my mother-in-law if she might like to come and live with us as soon as we'd found somewhere permanent. At the time, Rosie was living in a mobile home on the adjacent plot to her twin sister down by the water in Emsworth. It was lovely in summer, but had no heating and, never one to make a fuss, she'd seen in the previous New Year in bed with pneumonia without telling anyone.

Rosemary Turner – aka Granny Rosie – was a local girl born and bred. Growing up in Apuldram in the 1930s, one of the daughters of a gardener at the big house, she'd lived the kind of English rural childhood that no longer exists. Riding her beloved pony Minx to junior school and stabling her at her uncle's pub until going-home time, in 1941 Rosie took and passed the eleven-plus. After that, she cycled from her tiny village to the girls' grammar school in the city wearing her hated home-made uniform.

She did well – she was, as she put it, 'as clever as she was naughty' – so took her Higher School Certificate early. Left kicking her heels before she was old enough to start her teacher training, and needing to raise enough money to pay for the course, she spent the summer of 1947 giving rides on Minx. She worked in the fields of Apuldram and Dell Quay, singling sugar beet and stooking sheaves for 11d a day. Only a little more lucrative, in the autumn she was employed as a pupil teacher for £3 a month until she could take up her place. Each morning she'd present herself at County Hall in Chichester, to be sent anywhere in the district on her bicycle for a day's work.

In the forty-odd years between then and retirement, there'd been a long career as a teacher, three husbands who hadn't suited and three sons who did. As a consequence, she'd moved around a fair bit. Sometimes a little further west into Hampshire, sometimes further up into the Downs towards Midhurst, but always local.

Now unattached, and with no caring responsibilities of her own, in the summer of 1998 Rosie moved into our ramshackle house outside Bognor Regis – more building site than a home – bringing with her one or two favourite pieces of furniture, her electric keyboard, her books and music, but otherwise travelling light.

She was down to earth, unsentimental, used to fending for herself and a much-appreciated extra pair of hands for two working parents – the kind of granny who did cartwheels in the garden. If I was caught up at work, or my husband got stuck at the end of his teaching day, she stepped in. Standing *in loco parentis* at the gates of the same playground where my sisters and I had waited in the 1970s, and Rosie and her twin had lined up fifty years before that.

Small-town life.

The NHS gives the official definition of a carer as 'anyone, including children and adults, who looks after a family member, partner or friend who needs help because of their illness, frailty, disability, a mental health problem or an addiction and cannot cope without their support. The care they give is unpaid.'

All the same, it's a tricky word. It's a noun freighted with meaning and requiring qualification. It brings with it a hint of transaction, of an inequality, which is all the more uncomfortable if you're caring for someone you love. By using it, however accurate it might be in terms of the day-to-day realities, there's a risk that it redefines a partnership, a balanced give-and-take relationship, and turns it into an obligation: carer and patient, carer and client. One is active, the other passive, whereas every carer knows there's nearly always some kind of reciprocity even in the darkest hours.

You are still you, and they are still they.

More than a decade later, in the summer of 2009, my parents were to throw in their lot with us too.

A different house, in Chichester this time, it had been on the market for a while. Neglected and damp, with a strong smell of mould and stray cats, it had been a hostel, a home for nurses and, ironically, a care home. But it had a bright and airy single-storey annexe, previously a self-contained flat for the warden, which would suit my parents. Most significantly, it was wheelchair accessible – which was likely to matter a great deal in the years ahead as my father's Parkinson's became more severe.

This was the beginning of our two families and three generations living together under one roof – my husband and me, our teenage children, my 85-year-old father, my 77-year-old mother and my 78-year-old mother-in-law. For me, it was the beginning of becoming, and learning how to be, a carer, though each experience would be different: first, supporting my mother caring for my father, then holding a watching brief for her as she negotiated life without him. Finally, as a full-time extra pair of hands for Rosie. It's an odd role reversal – one that creeps up on you – when you realise that you are now caring for those who once cared for you.

And here we still live twelve years later – my husband Greg, Granny Rosie and I – with our companionship and our ghosts and our memories. In a house on the corner where three roads meet.

2

The House on the Corner

ALTHOUGH DIAGNOSED WITH PARKINSON'S DISEASE in his mid-seventies, my gentleman father, Richard Mosse, continued to live as himself – a retired cathedral-town solicitor, a member of the Rotary club and other local charities, a lay reader, a lover of the Sussex countryside, someone who enjoyed an occasional glass of white wine with lunch and a Glenmorangie before bed. A man of principle who enjoyed horse racing, *Ski Sunday* and Formula One.

But then, as so often in these narratives of ageing, there's a moment when the world stumbles, then falls.

Returning from a holiday in Spain in July 2004, a few weeks after his eightieth birthday, a virus caught on the plane sent my father into intensive care. Those anxious days were my first experience of what was to come. Sitting at his bedside in the ICU in the stifling heat of the afternoons, with motes of dust dancing in the air. Helping him to take sips of water, trying to ignore the wires and the remorseless bleep and hiss of the machines. Holding on tight to the hand that had once held mine.

Secure in his faith, he spoke of dying and of the lightness of letting go, but of how he wasn't yet ready to leave. And I, in that whispering voice peculiar to churches and waiting rooms, read aloud to him, stumbling my way through G. K. Chesterton's 'The Battle of Lepanto', one of his favourite poems from his schooldays: 'Dim drums throbbing, in the hills half heard ...' I wasn't sure he could hear me, but I was desperate to do something. Anything. Now, of course, I know that this sense of powerlessness, when watching someone you love struggle or suffer, is part and parcel of what it means to care.

Possibly to avoid my launching next into Tennyson's 'The Charge of the Light Brigade', he rallied. From the ICU, my father was moved onto the wards of the main hospital, where he stayed for several months. Doctors adjusting medications, nurses treating a secondary infection, it was a slow recovery. He was always courteous and uncomplaining, even though it still wasn't certain he would ever leave.

But on a wet afternoon in mid-October, he was transferred to the rehabilitation War Memorial Hospital nearby. A subdued place, a time-suspended place of hushed voices and empty corridors. The names of the men from our patch of Sussex who'd given their lives in two world wars were painted on a pale oak board in the lobby in gold leaf and black trim.

My father had joined up straight from school in 1942 and in 1943 was offered a commission in the 1st Battalion Welsh Guards. (For a brief and glorious moment, he was the youngest first lieutenant in the British Army.) He landed at Arromanches in Normandy, a few miles from Bayeux, on 25 June 1944, D-Day plus 19. He was part of the liberation of Brussels on 3 September and survived to return home. Others did not. Of three little boys who'd played together in the 1930s on the shingle at low tide in the new seaside parish of Aldwick, where my grandfather was vicar, only my father had come back. The names of his school friends, lost at the ages of eighteen and twenty-one, are recorded on that roll of honour in that quiet hospital hall.

In early November, on a day when the air was sharp with the smell of bonfires and damp earth, my father was finally discharged. Though he was still himself, the same sense of humour and warm twinkle in his eye, he had somehow aged many years in those four, treacherous months. It was clear that the Parkinson's had seen its chance and taken a firmer hold.

My parents' marriage had always been a partnership of equals, of respect, of shared purpose and interests. Well matched, contented, true. They'd celebrated their golden wedding the previous May in the company of their three daughters and eight grandchildren. Now, they were heading into uncharted waters.

Parkinson's is a degenerative condition, so although

my father was no longer ill, there were tiny declines: the trademark tremor in his left hand became a little more obvious, the stiffness in his muscles more limiting. Spring, summer, autumn and winter each year slightly more was lost. So many things previously taken for granted, some of the pleasures that distinguish an individual's life, had to be put aside or given up.

But not all.

My father's health improved and things returned, though at a slower pace, to almost normal. He was there to raise a glass to the publication of my novel, *Labyrinth*, the book that changed everything. He was there to welcome his first great-grandchild, he continued to enjoy meals out with friends and going to the theatre, he went racing at Goodwood and Fontwell, took gentle walks along the seafront. High days and anniversaries, a whisky nightcap at the end of the day, another Christmas, another birthday.

Life went on.

My mother never used the word 'carer' about herself, even though she was always there at my father's side when he needed her, believing that the word 'wife' contained multitudes. A vow taken on a glistening May afternoon in St Mary's Church, Ewell, in 1954, and kept.

But by 2009 – after a decision delayed and delayed again – it was accepted that my heroic mother was going to need more regular support, not least if she was to continue to live as herself. To be herself.

For many siblings, conversations about the next step

for ageing parents can be complicated and fraught with misunderstanding or grievance. What if they live in different parts of the country? What if parents need full-time, or part-time, care but won't accept help? Is sheltered or supported living more sensible? What's possible? Who's going to pay? Who might have the space, who might have the time, who does what? Independence, safety and proximity, everything has to be discussed and negotiated, especially in situations where a parent or parents are not able to make those decisions for themselves.

In many ways, it was easier for us than for lots of families – not least because there were no travel worries. Even though my parents were coming to live with us, it wouldn't make a difference to their relationships with anyone else. We three girls lived within spitting distance of one another anyway – and from where we'd grown up – we each saw our parents regularly and independently of one another, they knew and loved all of their grandchildren. My sisters had their own relationships with our mother and father, which adjusted over time as did mine. My parents moving to our house wouldn't change this. Greg and I were at a stage in our lives where we were flexible – we both worked from home – and we had time.

And we had, my sisters and I, a long and shared history.

I'm looking at a photograph of myself at the age of seven, hand on the tiller, on a boat on Fishbourne Creek. It's March, or maybe April, 1968. I'm not sure who owns the boat, but I'm wearing a peaked blue captain's hat, a thick white jersey and look half serious, half surprised at being in such a position of responsibility. I have never since been given command on the water ...

We grew up in Fishbourne in the 1960s and 70s, an old-fashioned Sussex village that hadn't changed so very much for generations. Our house was always full, a second home for other people's children. Even now, more than forty years later, so many of my friends can still remember the old telephone number off by heart. Silver birch trees in the front garden, yew trees along the back where the blackbirds made their nests, and a mighty laurel bush where my sisters and I made a camp out of sight of the dining-room window. When we were older, while loose-limbed boys sprawled and self-conscious girls sat chattering in the sitting room, my parents would be in the kitchen, talking with neighbours about local fundraising committees.

Just as important as our house was what lay beyond the village. Farmed fields to the west, the spire of Chichester Cathedral piercing the sky to the east. To the north, the green hills of the Sussex Downs. To the south, the mudflats and the reed mace that rattled like bones in the prevailing wind, and the sea.

Slipping out of the back door, along the cul-de-sac and across the main road. Walking faster now, down Mill Lane to the duck pond – where many generations of wellington boots came to the same muddy end – and at last out into the open where the Fishbourne Marshes lay spread out like an old map. I loved the old brooding Queen Anne house that sat – and sits still – at the head of the creek, looking out over the shifting expanse of water like a sentinel.

More often than not my sisters and I would take the right-hand path into the reedbeds and marram grass that towered over our heads. I loved the hushed stillness and the rills and streams that wound round and round. We would halt awhile on the middle of the three bridges to play Pooh sticks when the tide was high, before continuing on to the open fields and the estuary. We played *Swallows and Amazons* (without the boat) and Narnia (without the snow). We trekked single file along the old flint sea wall to what we called Oak Pond, where a scuttled rowing boat lay abandoned in the silted water.

Chill autumn days at dusk. Gulls and curlews shrieking out at sea and the hawthorn bushes stark and bare. Later, pinpricks of spring as the first wild flowers showed their colours in blossoms of blue and pink. The path across the estuary at low tide, with white markers showing the way across its muddy reaches. Lines of quivering poplar and ash. This was the real and remembered landscape of my childhood, both specific and timeless, one that gave me comfort when my father was dying. When he could no longer walk along the sea wall for himself, and my mother desperately needed to sleep, I'd fill the bleak hours between midnight and dawn with descriptions of what I'd seen that day: pale pink lady's smock; white traveller's joy; the blackthorn coming into flower; a sooty cormorant airing its wings, black-bellied dunlins flocking on the shore and sparrows in the hedgerows.

These are the memories I return to, time and again in the middle of another watchful night, on call in case something happens.

To care with love is not a transaction but, looking back at family photograph albums, with their faded colours and curled corners, one thing is clear. Though I didn't realise it at the time, throughout much of my childhood I was learning what it meant to care.

In their work lives and, just as significantly, their private lives, my parents made everyone welcome. Without fuss, they offered companionship and friendship in the spirit of community. They took responsibility, but never took over.

It's obvious, but it's worth saying: if you have a positive image of what it means to be interdependent – not dependent, nor wholly independent, but rather part of a reciprocal and ever-changing relationship of shared experiences, common memories, affection – it can be less difficult when and if the time comes for you to step up. It is much easier, much more possible, to be an extra pair of hands if you have been shown from the cradle how to do it.

3

Something Altogether Different

IN HER 2020 BOOK *Labours of Love,* a five-year investigation into the state of unpaid and paid care in the UK, Madeleine Bunting shares several derivations of that loaded little word.

First, from the Old English word *caru*, meaning anxiety, grief, sorrow; then from the Old German word *chara*, which translates as lament or a 'burden of the mind'. But also, from the Latin, *cura*. I prefer *cura*. It is less pessimistic in its definition of the give-and-take. It combines a sense of sadness, of burden, with the idea of attentiveness to another's welfare. Though its provenance is different, the modern Welsh word *caru* means 'to love'.

This paradox is at the heart of what it means to care – there are positives and negatives. Each one of us who finds ourselves in this position will have different emotions, at different times, and depending on our personal circumstances, our feelings for the person for whom we are asked to care, their needs and long-term situation, our own sense of what we are capable of giving and what we might have to sacrifice.

There is a deal of difference between being a carer and caring for someone in the normal run of things. There are plenty of acts of affection and support that we each undertake as part of our daily lives – be it cooking a meal, or popping round with shopping when a friend is ill, buying a present on behalf of someone else or making an appointment for them, picking up a neighbour's children at the end of school, or walking your sister's dog. Each of these, though important, are single acts of care, even if they are done regularly. They do not define you and your relationship. It's about being a good partner, a good neighbour, a good friend. The UK witnessed this during the early weeks of the first national lockdown in 2020 when more than a million people signed up to the NHS volunteer scheme.

There are lots of people who find themselves in between. They aren't full-time carers in this sense of being present every day. They might live a long way away. But, nonetheless, they are still wondering all the time how their parents are doing, are conscious of their health and happiness. It doesn't matter whether you are there or not, they will always be on your mind. There are many for whom the daily phone call to a loved one often raises more questions than it answers.

Being 'a carer' is something altogether different.

Whether you live with the person you're caring for or

not, being a carer is about every single day, sometimes about all the hours in every day. It's about routine, the endless repetition of things, of always having someone else's needs at the forefront of your mind. The quotidian tasks that repeat and repeat: conversations, medication, meals, laundry, personal hygiene. It's about the embracing of unpredictability and sudden change. It's about factoring in what is needed and when, and how it will be done. It is about thinking about someone else's food, someone else's needs for a newspaper or a doctor's appointment or a more comfortable position in which to sit. It is about having a parallel life running alongside your own. About never thinking of chucking everything up and walking out. And if there is a crisis in your own life which takes you out of the game, there must be a backup plan.

It's about thinking for two (or three or four) instead of one.

Practically, it's not unlike being a parent. Every new mother knows that you can't just have a shower when you fancy, but have to fit it around when your newborn baby is sleeping. You cannot act spontaneously. Every decision requires planning, even for those with a partner or family members at hand. But there's a crucial difference. All being well, the pattern of parenting is about your child growing stronger, more confident, more independent, learning to do things on their own and without your arms always there to catch them if things go wrong.

When caring for someone with a life-limiting illness or approaching the end of their life, it is de facto a journey in the opposite direction. When decline is inevitable – and it will come to us all – stability is the best one can hope for. It is how we manage this shift in emphasis that matters. Learning to live more slowly, to not be governed by the clock, to take pride and pleasure in ordinary things. It's hard.

Adapting or blending households, as we did, taking urgent calls in the middle of a meeting, changing arrangements to be available for a hospital appointment is becoming normal. So many of us now juggle caring responsibilities: the pressures of having to drive halfway across the county every weekend to visit parents who, though they might need support, quite understandably want to stay in their own homes, with their own friends nearby and their memories. It might be easier all round, but they don't want to be uprooted to live with their adult children. Or worrying about the lack of safe provision or the fear that their mother's or father's care home is not looking after them well enough. Or the mounting cost of things. Or trying to look after a sibling who can't manage on their own, but without the authority to step in.

Often it can feel as if there are no good options, only less bad ones.

Everyone's personal circumstances are unique and will be hugely influenced by their finances, their support networks, their housing, their own age and health, where they live, their ethnicity, the prejudices they face or the privileges they have.

Our situation changed out of the blue. A moment of

publishing good fortune in my mid-forties, when one of my novels became a bestseller, changed our lives. My husband Greg was a secondary school teacher. I went from working long hours in a theatre and writing in my spare time, to being a full-time author. It made all the difference to what we could manage to do, both in terms of our day-to-day availability and our resources. It made it easier to afford services and equipment the NHS couldn't provide. Later, as my father's condition worsened, it made it possible to be able to have paid carers in to help with some of the more intimate tasks.

For all carers, the pressures on time and finances are heavy. Many are obliged to give up their jobs for someone who needs round-the-clock care or support. Transport to and from hospital appointments, specialist equipment, laundry and respite care, all of this comes at a cost.

The burdens on young carers and sole carers, the challenges faced by those who are caring for more than one person, those caring for children or adults with long-term disabilities or additional needs, are even more extreme. Too often, the system fails to care for those who are caring for others. We saw this starkly during the pandemic. We should all be fighting for a higher standard of care for all of our older people, and those of any age who need additional support, so that dignity and choice are not simply a matter of postcode or family resources but rather built in to the heart of the system itself.

I suspect that anyone reading this book, regardless of

their own circumstances, will be grappling with similar questions: how best to be a 'good' daughter or son (or niece or sister, nephew or grandson); how to be a supportive sibling; how to distinguish between what you ought to do and what you feel capable of doing. As Caitlin Moran puts it in *More Than a Woman,* in middle age we are all aboard, or about to board, the 16.57 from London to Preston every Friday night to spend the weekend with a parent who needs support. In other words, my situation of finding myself a carer is common.

It can be distressing. Taking responsibility for another's needs may be willingly done and a privilege (it was, and is, for me), but there is a poignancy in the reality that someone who is visibly ageing and already fragile will only ever become less mobile, less able to manage. It's a tough gig, often full of despair and sadness. The nineteenth-century author Chateaubriand wrote: *la vieillesse est un naufrage* – old age is a shipwreck ... Granny Rosie has her own version: 'Getting old is not for the faint-hearted.'

Many carers talk about feeling guilty – that terrible disappointment on a beloved father's face when the visit is over too soon, or the falsely bright goodbye from a capable mother who is elderly herself, lonely as a sole carer, but refusing to give in. That wartime generation were brought up to cope, regardless of the personal consequences, rather than to ask for help. For many caring remotely, the constant questioning of whether or not you are doing the right thing, or doing it well enough, can be overwhelming, particularly for families where the pressures are already extreme on childcare or finances or their own ill health.

However much you do, it never feels enough.

But though often remorseless and exhausting, it's important also to celebrate the moments of caring that are rewarding and fulfilling, that are fun, however few and far between they might be. It's important to look for hope. Moments of love and engagement.

Because caring is all of these things. Shifting sands.

I'm remembering a visit to one of our favourite local pubs, a typical flint-faced Sussex cottage nestled in the green folds of Charlton Down. It was April 2010 perhaps, a year before my father died. One of his favourite authors, Rudyard Kipling, wrote: 'Smells are surer than sounds or sights/To make the heart-strings crack.' Certainly, I haven't forgotten the scent of polished wood, the aroma of herbs and meat roasting in the kitchen, the apple tint of local cider. I can see in my mind's eye, too, how my father, without any hint of self-pity, ordered a glass of red wine but asked for it to be served in two tumblers. Holding out his unstable hand to show how the tremors of Parkinson's made a full glass an accident waiting to happen.

'Do you see?' he said kindly, and they did.

Remembering, too, how my mother took these kinds of moments in her stride when it must have been painful to watch. She never spoke for him, never took over unless he wanted her help, never let the thing he could no longer do become more important than the things he could.

Moments of pride and admiration.

4

Women's Work?

CARERS UK ESTIMATE there could be as many as 8.8 million unpaid carers in the UK. That's one in six of the UK adult population who are involved in care of the long-term sick or elderly, a number that will shoot up in the next twenty years. Each year some 2.1 million adults take on unpaid caring responsibilities for an elderly or disabled relative – and, give or take, about the same number find their role as a carer coming to an end. Over a million carers are caring for more than one person. And the reality is that the biggest burden falls predominantly on daughters and daughters-in-law.

There are many sole carers, with no family support, and a distressingly growing number of young carers looking after parents or siblings – the Children's Society estimates there might be as many as 800,000 young people between the ages of 5 and 17 caring.

By the age of fifty-nine, women have a fifty–fifty chance

of being a carer. Men don't have equivalent odds until they are seventy-five. And these unpaid carers save the UK economy £132 billion per year. The carers allowance – for those who work over thirty-five hours a week – is £67.25 a week, in other words, £1.90 per hour. So very little.

There's a growing crisis in the paid sector too, where low pay is endemic and there are problems with recruitment and retention of staff. Here, too, the gender imbalance is just as clear: some 89 per cent of nurses are women, 75 per cent of social workers and 98 per cent of childcare professionals. By 2020, women formed the majority of GPs (54 per cent). In the NHS, some 80 per cent of healthcare workers and 82 per cent of social care workers for the long-term sick, disabled and frail elderly were women.

There's overwhelming evidence that Covid-19 has exacerbated the crisis in care and hugely impacted women's lives, particularly for black women, women of colour, those with fewer financial resources, and in areas of the country where investment in health and social services has been most savagely cut. In 2020, report after report gave evidence to how women were bearing the brunt of the economic shutdown. In May, a report from the Institute for Fiscal Studies and UCL Institute of Education revealed that mothers in England were more likely than fathers to have lost their jobs during lockdown. Amelia Hill in the *Guardian* in June estimated that an additional 4.5 million people – three times the size of the NHS workforce – were obliged to become unpaid carers for sick, older or disabled relatives because of the pandemic. In July, the management consultancy McKinsey reported figures showing that women were more vulnerable to Covid-19-related economic effects because of existing gender inequalities; in August, the *Lancet* published an article highlighting concerns; in September, the TUC warned that women were being 'pushed out of the workforce'; at the end of the year, after the second national lockdown in November, HRMC analysis showed that women were more likely than men to be 'let go' after the furlough scheme ended; and a survey carried out across the UK by a group of women's organisations, including the Fawcett Society, showed that 15 per cent of mothers – many of whom had caring responsibilities for an older family member too – had had to take unpaid time off from work compared with 8 per cent of fathers. Though full figures are not yet available, it's evident that for black and BAME communities the figures are likely to be even starker.

Care is a feminist issue.

Key in the strategy for care (or, rather, the lack of it) is the absence of women legislators, politicians, CEOs, policy makers. Those who have never taken the primary caring role in any situation are, clearly, less likely to understand what it means to care, how one juggles work and emotional responsibility. They are less likely to understand how their very lack of compassion and practical experience makes them unfit to be dictating policy.

This gender imbalance is one of the reasons, though by no means the only one, why the care industry, and caring as an unpaid profession, is so invisible, so ignored, so undervalued. As another magnificent octogenarian, the late Ruth Bader Ginsburg, put it: 'Women belong in places where decisions are being made.' In September 2020, at the beginning of the period of local tiered lockdowns when a second wave of Covid-19 was threatening, there was not a single woman at COBRA meetings. There was not a single nurse on the SAGE COBRA team. In mid-December, it was announced that, for the previous six months, every single No. 10 press briefing had been given by a man.

Women's work, but no women in the room.

In some ways, it's more challenging to be a carer if there are not already strong bonds of affection. Some women – and it is mostly women – find themselves caring for relatives they don't love or even particularly like, or to whom they have no reason to feel grateful. Stepfathers or stepmothers, aunts, mothers- or fathers-in-law. People who are irascible or self-centred, unkind or peevish. Neglectful. They find themselves responsible simply because there is no one else. Our overburdened care system relies on this, exploits this. And it's often those without children, or whose jobs are more accommodating, or who live closest to the person requiring care, who find themselves, willingly or unwillingly, having to take a bigger role.

Contemporary and classic literature is full of such relationships – in Agatha Christie's detective fiction there are many unmarried daughters whose lives have been sacrificed to the demands of tyrannical elderly fathers and armies of spinster sisters duty-bound to keep house for their widowed brothers. At the heart of P. D. James's *A Taste for Death* are two detectives whose working lives are compromised by the burden of caring for, or trying to avoid taking responsibility for, older relatives.

In the mid-nineteenth century, Charlotte Brönte was left alone – after the death of her mother, her aunt and her five siblings – in that rectory in Haworth caring for her formidable father. The mighty Ulster writer, Helen Waddell, was obliged to give up her hopes of going to Oxford University in 1912, after excelling as a scholar at Queens College, Belfast, because of the demands of her increasingly controlling, increasingly bullying stepmother. In an uncharacteristic moment of honesty about her difficult situation, Waddell wrote to a friend, Dr Taylor:

I got into the habit of never, unless for something tremendous, going out in the evenings. She [Martha Waddell] told me that my duty to her was as great as my duty to other people. There was no sacrifice she would not accept from me without so much as seeing it was sacrificed at all.

History matters, books matter. They entertain and illustrate and inform, they broaden our horizons. Novels, in particular, help us to process emotions and ideas, they enable us to stand in other people's shoes and reflect our own lived experience back at us. We can travel all over the world and through any period of time on the pages of a book. At the same time, I wonder if these literary and historical precedents of women being obliged to give up their dreams, expectations, ambitions in order to care for others, are still subconsciously shaping society's expectations now. That we still have a narrative of a woman's place being in the home not out in the world. As Adrienne Rich put it: 'a book of myths/in which/our names do not appear.'

Women's stories ...

5

An Indian Summer

IT IS AUGUST 2009 WHEN my PARENTS finally move into the annexe. The old carpets had gone, Ma had chosen her favourite colours for cupboards, worktops and blinds, it was light and accessible.

As the afternoon shadows dance on the lawn, we three girls carry and unpack boxes, arrange crockery in their new kitchen, shuffle pieces of furniture about until they find their perfect spot: the mahogany glass-fronted dresser, filled with commemorative plates and cut-glass decanters; the inlaid beech card table, the old tapestry fire screen, the two-tiered oak bookcase that used to stand at the top of the stairs holding my father's treasured copy of *The Rubaiyat of Omar Khayyam*, a fond memento of his army posting to Palestine in 1946; my mother's library of glossy coffee-table books celebrating the Hollywood golden years and MGM musicals.

My parents had downsized twenty years earlier, when

moving from our childhood home in Fishbourne, but, even so, there is a great deal to fit in. My sisters and I help to hang up clothes and put shoes away, find a corner by the front door for my father's collection of walking sticks, stack my mother's computer and box files on the wide white shelves built for the purpose, abandon rogue paperwork on the dining table. Posters and mementos from my father's time in the theatre – after being demobbed in 1948, he'd been an actor-manager before deciding to train as a solicitor. My husband drills and hammers and taps, hanging pictures on their new walls and adjusting curtain rails.

Too often, we get distracted by the cumbersome old photograph albums. The rustle of waxed paper, the scent of dust and family history preserved: Ma at eighteen with her beloved dog Pip, looking like a young Elizabeth Taylor; a seaside snap of her with her mother and younger brother Christopher, her black curly hair framing her face; my father in 1947 in the heat of the Jordanian desert in his army uniform holding a Bakelite telephone in his right hand like a stage prop; their honeymoon in Guernsey in 1954; my sisters and I having a picnic in the 1960s. Weddings and christenings. A colourful record of their travelling years in their early sixties when retired and free of child-rearing responsibilities. Vivid, bright images full of life.

And some photos we've never seen before: a joyous one of Ma's retirement from the local branch of Scope, surrounded by flowers and well-wishers; another to honour her work for the Citizens Advice Bureau; her final cohort of students at Chichester College; my father's bowling group; Ma's astonished expression at her surprise sixtieth birthday party.

Finally, all the boxes have been brought in from the van. The unpacking is almost done. Everything has found a place. The sun is still shining and will keep shining for another fortnight into September.

An Indian summer.

But soon, there's a hint of copper and gold on the leaves, starlings chattering in the neighbour's sweet chestnut tree. We're on the cusp of autumn. Filigree spiders' webs glisten with dew in the early morning.

During those first weeks as next-door neighbours, we settled into a routine.

My mother popping in for coffee; my father taking a gentle stroll up and down the garden most afternoons, often followed by the ever-hopeful dog thinking this might be a second walk. Ma kneeling with trowel and gloves, preparing her flowerbeds for winter bedding plants. Reds and yellows to keep the grey of the cold months at bay.

All the change-of-address cards have been dispatched. The myriad adjustments made to living somewhere new were accomplished – doctors' surgery, bank, telephone, my mother's driving licence, tick, tick, tick and tick. She continued as secretary to the governors at the primary school in Felpham. My father continued to see friends from his Freemason days. Though there's always been a deal of criticism and uncomfortable talk about Freemasonry, for him it was a place of comradeship and faith and tradition, a community that linked him to his father and his father before him. His Parkinson's medication was, for the most part, keeping the worst of his symptoms under control. He seemed well. And if there might be a problem, we were right next door. They went every Sunday to my youngest sister for lunch, went on outings with their grandchildren.

Their lives had found a new pattern.

When not knitting or dog walking for neighbours, Granny Rosie was performing in local care homes with her entertainment troupe, playing a programme of old musical hall songs and World War II favourites. Her electric keyboard with its collapsible legs lived permanently in the boot of her car, ready for the next gig.

Two independent households, but living side by side and, notwithstanding the usual niggles in any cheek-by-jowl family, we rubbed along happily enough.

Three generations living together – it seemed to work.

And there seemed to be more time to talk.

Not the snatched 'how are you?' on the phone or a quick cup of tea in the blue hour of the fading afternoon, but to talk properly. Time enough for a glass of wine when the sun was over the yard arm. All carers know the pressure when you have to leave. The sense that, however long you stay, it will never be quite long enough. We escaped that.

If my father fancied a little company when Ma was out, I'd coax out of him stories about his childhood, though he never much liked talking about himself. He preferred to listen.

He was the youngest child of the Reverend Charles Herbert Mosse and Beatrice (Betty) Elizabeth Mosse, née Watson. They'd married at Streatham Hill in September 1918, when Granddad was home on leave from his position as an army chaplain. After the war, he continued his ministry, first in London and then in Horsham, West Sussex. It was, as my father put it, a happy and uneventful childhood until he was six.

Every summer, the family decamped to Newlands Valley in the Lake District, in the shadow of Causey Pike. They drank unpasteurised milk bought directly from a local farm and, in those days, herds were not routinely tested. One morning, my father complained to Granny about having a headache. She took his temperature and, though very much of the stiff-upper-lip generation, was alarmed and sent his older sister Margie to fetch the doctor from further down the valley. No car, no telephone, no time to borrow the farmer's horse-and-trap, just a worried young girl running as fast as she could to get help. The diagnosis was pulmonary TB.

At this point in the story, my father would smile. 'So I was sent to bed,' he'd say, 'and there I stayed for a year ...'

Nothing could be done to accelerate his recovery. Just rest and, above all, fresh air. So, in 1931, my grandfather left Horsham for the south coast to become the first vicar of the new parish of Aldwick. And rather than going back to school with his older brother, my father remained at home in the vicarage with his mother and sister for company, confined first to bed, then into a bath chair, then gradually learning to walk again. One of the lucky ones, he recovered, though it was not until two years later that he was back in the Lake District and strong enough to attempt Causey Pike.

It was in that same whitewashed house in Newlands Valley in 1939 that the family sat silent, around the wireless at eleven o'clock on 3 September, to hear the prime minister, Neville Chamberlain, announce that Great Britain was now at war with Germany.

Although Ma was always dashing about, she had her stories too.

Born Barbara Towlson, in the shadow of the Woolwich Arsenal in south-east London, she was an outstanding student at school – I have inherited some of her old subject reports. The war interrupted her education, as it did for so many children. She endured an unhappy evacuation to Wales with her mother and little brother, then a happier one in Yorkshire. When they finally came back to bomb-damaged London, she had to give up her hopes of a place at university in order to take a job and contribute to the family finances. Instead of dreaming spires and lecture halls, she trained as a shorthand typist and achieved crazy fast speeds. She was snapped up by a legal firm in central London, where she met a former captain in the Welsh Guards, who was now training to be a solicitor after a few years in the theatre. 'Your father,' she'd add, in case of doubt, and we'd giggle.

Ma never talked as if she felt she had missed out, or with regret about opportunities she hadn't been able to take. But despite everything she achieved in her life, I know she would have triumphed at university and they would have been lucky to have her.

It is a great gift to have time to get to know your parents as people. As the selves they were before they were your mother and father.

6

The Blue Light

NOVEMBER 2009.

My memories of the afternoon it happened are blurred, frayed around the edges. I can only remember that, coming home from their regular Sunday-lunch date with my youngest sister, my father tripped as he came through the gate and fell heavily, hitting his head. The dog barking, blood on the paving stones, my father's disappointed eyes and my mother's distraught face. Shouting. Doors opening and closing. Footsteps.

My footsteps?

I can remember dialling the emergency services and hearing a calm voice at the end of the line promising that help was on its way. I can remember whispering dishonest reassurances over and over that everything was going to be all right. A form of praying, perhaps. Fetching blankets to keep them warm and a pillow for my father's head. Holding my mother's hand. Watching and waiting and waiting.

These are actual memories, honest fragments. But it was only afterwards that I put them into some kind of order. A logical sequence of actions and reactions because ... well, that is how it must have been. At the time, everything seemed to happen simultaneously. And the truth is that each significant moment of decline or trauma comes accompanied with very similar emotions: disbelief, fear, indecision, urgency, powerlessness, panic, sympathy, pity. For although this was the first time the ambulance was called to our house on the corner, it was very far from being the last.

Finally, the siren and the blue light.

Is it to protect our tattered hearts from too much pain that we only half remember? That we hold on to certain tiny details, vivid and sharp, but let the broader picture drift out of focus?

So many snapshots of being in the hospital – that peculiar washed-out light, the pale blue curtains, metal-framed beds and high-backed regulation chairs, the organised chaos of A&E. Charts and questions, name and date of birth repeated until the words lose any meaning, blood pressure and lists of medication to be shared. The squeak of rubber-soled shoes as nurses and doctors and paramedics come and go, as if in a dance where we, the outsiders, have not been taught the steps.

The real world of saving lives is nothing like *Grey's Anatomy*. There are no familiar faces, no set-up, climax and resolution, no clear narrative. Just strangers and waiting with the desperate hope that, soon, someone will come with answers and solutions – not more questions.

Looking back, I simply can't remember. Did I go to the hospital with my mother in the ambulance or follow on? Was it me who called my sisters or my husband? Was my father kept in triage in A&E for twenty minutes or for many hours? I do have a memory of him looking vaguely concerned, rather than frightened, perhaps by the idea he was being a nuisance. I know that I realised he was oddly less worried for himself than for my mother. Or that might have been another occasion in A&E. Even in the most challenging of circumstances, people do not change essentially. My father was courteous, quietly grateful for the care he was being given, even when it was intrusive or undignified, and always remained so.

It was touch and go. The next weeks were distressing, frightening and exhausting for my mother. For us all. The same five-minute drive to the hospital each day and the inevitable ten-minute battle to find a parking space. The same discussions with doctors about what, if any, the longer-term damage might be. The same circular negotiations over treatment. The unfailing kindness of the nurses. The same corridors smelling of disinfectant and resignation.

A month passed and, against all expectation, my father recovered enough to be discharged home in the middle of a winter that seemed particularly long and dark.

It was a reprieve but, as before, the trauma had exacerbated my father's Parkinson's symptoms. As well as tremors and 'freezing' – when the body simply won't do what the brain is telling it – other symptoms began to show themselves. The dyskinesia, a side effect of medication that causes involuntary movements, was worse. The fear of falling made him anxious. He could no longer walk far unaided, so he needed a wheelchair. We acquired an electric reclining chair and a higher bed with a special mattress; we found lights that could be activated by the slightest touch of the hand. These were minor adjustments in the scheme of things, but it all helped.

It mattered, though. The aesthetics matter. Our NHS is amazing in the support and equipment it provides, but no one wants their house to look like a hospital ward. If possible, home needs to look like home.

Looking back with hindsight, I realise how I have lived my life surrounded by older people – my paternal grandmother died when she was ninety-one, my maternal granny (who lived round the corner from us in Fishbourne and then in Felpham) was ninety-eight, and my godmother Sister Katherine Maryel, an Anglican nun, died in 2016 at the age of 104. I'd been raised to believe that it wasn't a person's age that made them a good companion but rather what they did, how they lived alongside others. Nine years old or ninety, it was a person's character that mattered.

Too often old age is presented as a problem to be solved, when it should be a cause for celebration that many women and men are living enjoyable, contented, valued and beloved lives well into their eighties and nineties. The language around ageing needs to change from negative to positive, from something seen as a regrettable challenge to a sign of success.

Of course there are consequences of people living into their ninth, even their tenth or eleventh decade. First, the issue of quality of life. Improved life expectancy matters, yes, but so does living well and with dignity. Put simply, our bodies wear out with the passing of the years, regardless of whether or not we have some life-limiting or life-restraining illness.

Second, the issue of who does the caring. What about those who are alone? What about those women and men who are estranged from their families, or have no families to be estranged from? Or those who have no money for paid care? How do we support carers who have health problems of their own? Many women are called upon to become carers when they are struggling with the worst symptoms of the menopause, or still have child caring responsibilities, or possibly the onset of health problems of their own. What about carers who are elderly themselves? These are huge challenges.

For those with the devastating responsibility of looking after someone suffering from dementia or Alzheimer's things are exponentially harder. Rachel Mills's *Fragments of my Father*, Grace Dent's *Hungry*, about the onset of her father's dementia, and Nicci Gerrard's *What Dementia Teaches Us About Love* detail quite how tough it can be. Some 81 per cent of carers say they feel lonely or socially isolated and some 40 per cent have had to cut back on food and heating to make ends meet. Research from Carers UK in 2020 revealed that 72 per cent of carers suffered difficulties with their own mental ill health and 61 per cent reported physical ill health.

The Dilnot Commission on the Funding of Care and Support was set up in 2010, reported in 2011, the paper was ratified by Parliament and the Queen in 2015, then derailed by party politics. Ten years since its foundation, still none of the Commission's recommendations have been implemented. This lack of action, especially given the challenges so many carers are facing in the times of Covid – and after a year of isolation – is unforgivable.

On a day-to-day level, a change of both the language of ageing and attitudes expressed about it can make an immediate difference. Long-term illness is a struggle, it shrinks a person's world. There is a letting go of many of the issues that once seemed so important. Most people do not become any less themselves as they age or their health fails. My father remained my father – gentle, considerate, accepting.

By the spring of 2010, paid carers were coming in for half an hour, twice a day, to help with the more intimate and physically demanding aspects of getting up in the morning and going to bed at night.

My father's hands were less obedient, making eating and drinking less pleasurable, and he was suffering from dysphagia, a disruption to the swallowing process. My middle sister bought him a silver straw so he could sip his wine elegantly. My husband bought packs of rubber accountant's thimbles, which lived in a pot on the kitchen table, so he could still turn the pages of his newspaper at breakfast in the mornings. In the afternoons in June and July, when the weather was fine, he and I would take a spin around the block in his wheelchair. Even though the spasms in his neck were uncomfortable and unsightly, he never failed to raise his hat to anyone we met who was, like us, out taking the air. We watched houses being extended and rebuilt, the blossom trees coming into flower in adjacent roads, the shadows getting longer as the sun rose higher in the sky.

Life breathed and stretched, shifted its shape again, and went on.

My parents were now great-grandparents for a second time; I was struggling with a new novel; my husband was teaching; Granny Rosie celebrated her eightieth birthday; our almost grown-up children came and went and came back again, filling the house with their friends and, sometimes, with their absence.

All this time, through the summer and autumn of 2010 and then in the approach to Christmas, my mother did her best to remain positive though it took its toll. She was determined to remain out in the world, despite having a few of her own health issues to deal with. She had been born with a small hole in her heart, corrected by an operation in 2003. Ma took blood-thinning medicine, warfarin, so weekly blood tests were the order of the day, and she also had COPD. She was still an Embassy girl, while my father had been a Dunhill smoker until he'd given up twenty years earlier under doctor's advice.

Nonetheless, though she was very tired and worn down by the endless nature of things, she never failed to provide a listening ear for a friend or neighbour or to offer practical advice, if required.

But it's easier to give advice than to take it.

Sitting in the garden, Ma and I would talk about how important it was that carers – even if she still didn't think of herself in that way – were kind to themselves too. How they should accept that, sometimes, they'd feel snappy or ill, be frustrated or resentful of the time spent in the hospital or clinic. That this was normal. That this was just what it meant to be human. A wonderful, generous, compassionate human trying one's best and occasionally falling short.

I felt I was falling short most of the time. It was easy to sit with my father, peaceful even. But I felt I wasn't doing enough to look after my mother. I was impatient sometimes and frustrated. All carers, or supporters of carers, know that it takes a great deal of effort and stamina to take each day as it comes. To stay optimistic. To allow time to pass in the way it has to. Things cannot be rushed. Routine, repetition, regularity. Things take as long as they take.

7

The Uncertain Hour

YOU GET USED TO NOT SLEEPING. At least, to never sleeping properly. Too many things can go wrong in the night. So, although you go to bed and turn out the light, you remain alert. The bedroom door ajar, your mobile phone on your bedside table, just in case.

Always listening.

For any parent, this is familiar territory. From the instant you hold your baby in your arms, that twisting fear in your gut that something will happen while you're momentarily distracted never goes away. Putting your fingers under their tiny nose in the middle of the night to make sure they're still breathing, it's a kind of hyper vigilance that makes us ready to defend, launch into action, protect. Years later, we lie awake in bed listening for the front door to close, the stumble of teenage footsteps on the stairs. They're later than agreed, but never mind. They are safely home.

And breathe.

It's different at the other end of the story. For an older person with long-term health problems – breathing, mobility, pain – the simplest stumble might lead to something serious. Falling out of bed in the dark, the need for the bathroom, a wild nightmare brought on by the cocktail of essential medication with horrifying side effects. And for those with dementia or Alzheimer's, the confusion of the day might be compounded by the darkness or being lost in a world where time no longer exists. It is awful for those who love them to have to witness.

Night terrors.

Everyone who has a watching brief for someone else, whether you live together or not, knows the lurch in the pit of your stomach when the phone begins to ring at 4 a.m.

In September 1981, Ma and I had gone to Egypt on holiday on a whim.

A few weeks before I was due to head off to university, my mother realised I was rather low and decided a change of scene would help. I was twenty, at the end of a lonely gap year where I'd worked in a local cafe, done a secretarial course in London, temped as a secretary and made no friends. Listening to Ultravox and Phil Collins on a loop and with self-pity, or Janis Ian and Carole King, I'd gone home to Sussex miserable most weekends. In a flurry of travel agents' brochures and purpose, she booked us on a package tour leaving in four days' time.

Our tour group was, for the most part, made up of retired English travellers (and one middle-aged woman hoping to find the man with whom she had fallen in love twenty years before). I was the baby of the group; Ma was the life and soul.

After a few days in Cairo, we flew south to Karnak and stayed in a hotel in Luxor. It lives in my mind as a white and golden palace, beautiful and elegantly fading. Terraces with palm trees overlooking the Nile.

Venturing out before the worst of the heat flattened all colour and spirit from the day, we set off in a bone-rattling coach to visit the Valley of the Kings. In the long, sloping entrance corridor to one of the tombs – I think it was KV 11, the Tomb of Ramses III – was an exquisite fresco of the passage of the sun through its twenty-four-hour cycle. At three in the morning, a snake swallows the sun completely.

Huddled in the sombre light and dust of that ancient passage, I listened as the guide explained how the human spirit was at its most vulnerable between three and six in the morning. Those were the darkest hours, when spirits were at their lowest and when every sound, every thought, every emotion was amplified. Six weeks shy of my twenty-first birthday, I had no idea what it was like to be always watchful and awake and anxious as the dawn approached. To be, as T. S. Eliot's 'Little Gidding' puts it,'In the uncertain hour before the morning/Near the ending of interminable night.'

I do now.

Several times in these past twelve years, I've remembered my naive younger self in that tomb in Egypt. And found comfort in how, despite the passing of time and the millennia of information, knowledge and progress, the ebbs and flows of human emotion remain the same down the centuries. The ancient Egyptians knew. And we know that those dark tipping hours in the middle of the night are the hardest. It's then that self-pity and despair, doubts and regrets and anxiety creep in.

It leaves a scar.

It had been a good Christmas, in spite of everything. We'd had a small party on Christmas Eve. Ma had worn a beautiful black woollen dress and I vividly remember my father smiling as he made his goodbyes, waving his white handkerchief to the assembled company. It was a trick he'd developed to disguise his tremor, knowing how people found it distressing to see.

The January of 2011 came in cold and damp and, with it, the sense of something about to happen. My father's Parkinson's was no worse, yet he was plagued with additional problems: secondary infections of one kind or another that refused to respond to treatment, or fought with his medication. More intrusive tests and visits to the doctors' surgery meant that nothing was sitting well.

Too many hospital visits.

Every one of us mindful of elderly parents, or who cares for someone with a life-limiting condition, is alert to the tiny incremental changes that might mean something bigger is going on. In his poem 'Lines to Dr Walter Birk on his Retiring from General Practice', W. H. Auden suggests that a good doctor is one who can understand 'what our bodies are trying to say'.

Carers can do this too, hyper aware of the slightest variation in skin colour, or that the eyes are dulled or set too far back in their sockets. Concern can lead to an annoying number of repetitive questions: 'Are you all right ...?' 'Are you sure you don't need to ...?' 'Have you taken ...?' Though done for the best of reasons – not least of all, hoping to catch any medical problem that might be brewing in good time – the result can create an atmosphere of everything being about illness or decline. Sometimes, it's just better to shut up. Not always put someone's symptoms or their illness centre stage.

In February, after another afternoon spent being prodded and poked, my father said quietly under his breath as we were wheeling the chair back to the car: 'This is really becoming too much.' He was clear-sighted and without a shred of pity. With my mother's help – and ours, too – he had been managing his symptoms and his illness for years. But he was right.

In March and April, my father had a sequence of transient ischemic attacks – or TIAs as they're known – like mini strokes. Each one was distressing, undignified and exhausting for him and for my mother. It was an unequal battle between his zest for life and a body that was failing.

There are a range of symptoms and those who suffer

with Parkinson's – and it is a suffering – won't have them all. But my father now developed anosmia, a loss of smell, which meant that what little pleasure remained in eating – his hands now shook so much – was lost. And he slept very badly, often waking two or three times during the night. My mother had promised, as had I, that he would die at home, but it was taking a huge toll on her. When she needed a proper night's rest, Greg or I, or sometimes my youngest sister's husband, would sit with him in Ma's place, watching the hands of the clock move round and listening to the sighing movement of the special NHS mattress.

Waiting for the dawn.

There are so many gadgets designed to help older people or those with physical limitations of one kind or another: things to help you grip, to reach, to balance, to carry. Some are more effective than others, but they all, in the end, merely offer interim solutions to problems that cannot be fixed. If you have no strength left in your fingers, or your hands, then no device or gadget will help. And when that happens, it's another disappointment. Another tiny loss of independence.

It was becoming too much.

We talked a lot during these final weeks of his life, my father and I.

I sensed in him a liberation that came with the acceptance that his life was drawing to its end. Memories, reflections he'd never before wanted to share. He talked for the first time of his darker wartime experiences: about the poison of collaboration and how he witnessed it dividing French families; about the mud and confusion of Normandy; about his commanding officer being shot dead beside him; about the friends who didn't make it; about being showered with flowers and champagne as his battalion came into Brussels in September 1944, before being fired upon by snipers hiding in the burnt-out buildings. He talked of the shock of seeing the first images in the newspapers of the Nazi concentration camps. Shadows and lost friends, like the names on the memorial board in the rehabilitation hospital in Bognor.

For anyone of my parents' generation, the war is always there in the background. It was the backdrop to their formative experiences as children or as teenagers; it shaped their emotions, their characters, their sense of safety and of self. As he talked, I marvelled at their resilience, that determination to get on with things and not make a fuss, their resolve to suffer ill health without complaint.

I was working on a novel – set during World War II, in fact – but I found it hard to concentrate. My father's ghosts and my imaginary characters fought for space in my mind. Usually, my writing thoughts are sharpest just before it gets light, at those liminal moments between sleep and waking when my imagination is uninterrupted by the matters of a normal day: feeding the dog, making breakfast for others, emptying the dishwasher, remembering that it's bin day (again). Hearing the first song of the blackbird, seeing the silhouettes of trees coming back into focus, watching the splintering of the black into layers of blue, then white, pink and orange. The shepherd's warning.

That spring, I don't think I slept all the way through an entire night. The truth is – as all carers know – that it's never just the one night that grinds you down, but all of them set head to toe. Like dominoes falling. The cumulative effect of never sleeping properly plays havoc with your state of mind, makes everything fuzzy around the edges. Endless cups of sweet tea and biscuits. Too much coffee jangling your nerves, Prufrock's spoons measuring out the passing of time. Physical tasks, practical tasks, are mostly doable, give or take. They are easier to fulfil. But the imagination takes a bashing. Everything is dulled by exhaustion and sadness. Looking back, I can't believe I even tried to keep writing, but it gave a purpose to the days and the nights. It gave the illusion of some kind of control.

These challenges are complicated for the person for whom you are caring too. Most older people do not want, in Granny Rosie's words, 'to be a trouble'. Sometimes, they won't call for help because they're aware (and this is the situation for many carers) that their carer has additional caring demands, a full-time job, pressures on their own health, children. The list goes on. It's easier said than done, I know, but it's another reason why, even in those days where you want to do nothing but cry or shake your fists at the unfairness of it all, talking about caring in hopeful and positive terms matters. Trying to stay optimistic whatever the daily reality. It's an act of kindness for those who are being cared for not to focus only on the tough stuff, so they don't feel guilty for being a burden.

This hierarchy of care, deciding whose needs must come first, is something we have to negotiate. All carers know the nagging fear of not doing anything quite well enough. Of not being present enough for the other people in our lives. Friendships can fall away, neglected. It's not intentional, but there are only so many hours in the day.

I couldn't have done it without my husband. Greg was strong enough to physically support my father when his coordination let him down or if he needed help with personal things. Always sensitive to my father's needs, Greg cared with no fuss, no embarrassment, remained steady and calm. He looked after me, so that I could look after my parents.

Besides, what did it matter if I wasn't sleeping? Compared to most, I was in a hugely privileged position. Working from home, no longer having to do the school run, no need to be bright-eyed at a desk in the outside world each morning. But that low-level exhaustion rubs away at your stamina. And my anticipated grief at the loss I knew was coming leaked into everything, including the pages of the novel I was supposed to be finishing. The real world was casting a shadow over the imagined one.

It's hard to write when your heart is breaking.

Friday 29 April 2011 was a perfect spring day, sunny and warm, without being hot. A light breeze lifted the silver underside of leaves on the trees outside our front door.

Our neighbours were planning a street party to celebrate the marriage of Kate Middleton to Prince William. All morning, tables and chairs were being carried out into the road and set up. A marquee had been pitched in someone's front garden, waiting for the moment the food and drink would be brought out after the broadcast of the wedding was over.

We all went. My husband and I, my parents and Granny Rosie. My mother was in her element, elegant in red, white and blue. Granny Rosie had knitted a woollen queen and corgis to put around a straw bonnet. My father made a huge effort to put on a jacket, shirt and tie rather than the more casual clothes that were easier, now, to manage. His straw hat. Courteously refusing any food or drink as too complicated to negotiate, but smiling and part of things. Listening and being out in the world with the sun on his face.

Did I know at the time that it might be the last public thing my father would ever do? Probably not. But the memory of the dappled light and the glasses raised in a toast, the high spirits and camaraderie, are finely drawn in my mind. I am thankful for the memory of that afternoon. And when we returned home, all of us together, I remember feeling so grateful that we could still have such days.

8

The Undiscovered Country

IT IS MAY 2011, and my father is dying. My gentle, honourable father is dying.

A Monday afternoon. My parents' bedroom is full of afternoon light and dappled sun filtering through the sweet chestnut tree. The GP has come and gone, promising to return on Wednesday – or earlier, if need be. He's a doctor of the old school, the days of home visits and taking the time to get to know his patients. Though most people say they would like to die at home, only one in five of us get our wish. My mother promised my father that he would die in his own bed and, thanks to our compassionate and supportive local surgery and NHS doctors and nurses, he will.

It's peaceful in this room now, quiet and ordered. The shallow rise and fall of my father's chest, the sound of a blackbird grumbling at rooks in the garden, a neighbour mowing their lawn. The road is busy outside, on the far side of the fence. Other people on the school run. It seems extraordinary – wrong – that normal life is carrying on.

The ticking of the clock on my father's bedside table and his watch beside it, too heavy now for his thin wrist. Sounds of my mother in her kitchen and, beyond the party wall, the echo of footsteps on the tiled floor of our kitchen. Rosie is in the garden. I suspect she's keeping out of the way, not thinking she has the right to be here, but she's family too and her face is drawn.

An ordinary afternoon in May, the prettiest of months. Colourful and hopeful, a green-and-white month. My parents married in May. In the wedding photograph I have on a shelf in my study – they are looking at one another, not to the camera. My father has a carnation in his buttonhole, my mother a bouquet of springtime blooms.

My father's favourite flowers are bluebells. Every year, when my sisters and I were little, we'd go walking in the ancient bluebell woods of West Stoke and Goodwood, picking our way in March and April through the purple seas in single file. Now, those flowers have faded and, in any case, it's been a while since he's been able to leave the house. But if he were to open his eyes, he would still see the petals of the yellow roses in the border my mother planted, the earliest red flowers of the camellia.

My father is dying.

Over the past few weeks, there have been several false alarms, but we all know this is it. He is lying very still. The terrible Parkinson's spasms that distorted his neck, his shoulders and his hands have released him now and he seems peaceful, as if this were simply sleep. It's only the ragged breathing that gives it away.

The gaps between each inhalation grow longer.

For several days, we have been coming and going: my husband and I, our children, my sisters and their families, dear Granny Rosie. My father and Rosie have become good friends. Every Monday, when Ma goes to do the supermarket shop and have a sneaky coffee with friends, she's gone in with her knitting and they've spent the morning in companionable silence, or watching *Bargain Hunt*. It always touched Rosie that, whatever time Ma came home – even if it was just before the final minutes of the show when all would be revealed – he would turn off the television to ask her how her morning had been.

All of us, in our different ways, have been saying our goodbyes, even though we're still somehow hoping such leave-takings are premature. They have been before. To lose a parent is in the natural order of things. Children should outlive their parents. All the same, I'm not ready.

I've always disliked the euphemisms used to avoid saying the words 'death' and 'dying'. Phrases like 'passing on' or 'slipped away' or 'gone' always seemed mealy-mouthed and dishonest. But now, as I sit here, 'passing on' seems an accurate, even a lovely, description. Passing from this world to, as Hamlet says, 'the undiscovered country from whose bourn no traveller returns'.

*

Though it upset my mother, my father wanted to discuss the music and readings for his funeral service. In particular, the prayers he wanted and the hymns, the fragments of poems. As a young man, he'd kept a notebook recording favourite verses and lines, and he had returned to those yellowing pages now.

The list was typed – so despite her misgivings, Ma must have done this for him – together with brief explanations of why each had been chosen: Hymn 375, 'Lord of the Dance', because 'it is a happy hymn', and Hymn 368, 'Guide Me, Oh, thou Great Redeemer' to the tune of Cwm Rhondda, to honour his wartime experiences with the Welsh Guards. The word 'happy' appears several times on the list and that gave me comfort.

And between reciting familiar prayers and receiving his final sacrament, he talked with joy and anticipation at the promise of seeing his beloved mother again, his father and his brother, of being reunited with the men who died beside him on that beach in Arromanches. Of seeing God.

Despite his experiences in the ICU seven years previously, it was only now that I fully understood his profound belief meant he was certain he was on the cusp of a new adventure. He had no fear, no regrets – except for leaving my mother – no sense of having been cheated. Acceptance and grace. His life exemplified the sentiment of the nineteenth-century writer Étienne de Grellet du Mabillier, words that he asked to be printed on the inside front cover of the order of service:

I expect to pass through this world but once;
any good thing therefore that I can do,
or any kindness that I can show to any fellow human being,
let me do it now; let me not defer or neglect it,
for I shall not pass this way again.

My father died peacefully in his sleep on the afternoon of Wednesday 18 May, twelve days before his eighty-seventh birthday. He died in his own bed, as he'd wished, and with his family around him.

After it was over, and before all the formalities began – with the doctor and the undertaker – we remained there for an hour or so, in the sweet light of the afternoon, talking quietly around the bed, as if he was still with us: 'And flights of angels sing thee to thy rest.'

His funeral takes place on a beautiful summer's day in June at their old parish church in Felpham.

The building is packed to the rafters. My father was someone who people liked and respected. A true gentleman, is the phrase they use. People from all chapters of his long life are here – his brother Freemasons, all the societies and charities he'd supported over a lifetime of giving, carers who looked after him in the past six months, colleagues from his old firm of solicitors and the theatre, school friends of my sisters and mine, neighbours of more recent acquaintance.

Greg, our daughter Martha and our son Felix are there beside me, making sure I'm all right. My father had given

Felix his signet ring a few weeks earlier and he has it in his pocket. The doors are kept open and I can hear a robin singing in the graveyard outside.

My mother is poised and strong in her grief. Later, she will say a few perfect words in the church hall next door that will summon up the spirit and the character of her husband. My youngest sister and our cousin read together from the Book of Revelation; my father's oldest surviving friend gives the eulogy; I stumble through the closing lines of 'Little Gidding'; and my aunt, the same beloved older sister who ran pell-mell to fetch the doctor in Newlands Valley eighty years ago, delivers the prayers from her wheelchair. Now in her nineties, she was one of the first women to be ordained into the Anglican Church and my father was very proud of that.

As the prayers come to an end, we all get to our feet. I can still hear the robin singing. And when we raise our grieving voices to sing 'Lord of the Dance', the vaulted ceiling of the church is filled with sound.

My father was right. It is a happy hymn. His final gift to all of us left behind.

Richard Hugh Mosse
30 May 1924 – 18 May 2011

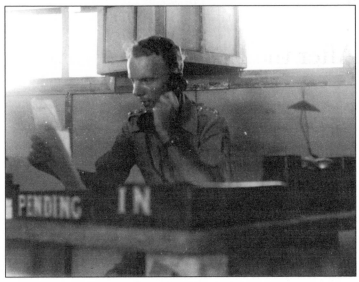

Captain Richard Mosse, Jordan, 1947

9

After the Funeral

BETWEEN THE DYING and the laying to rest, the heart goes into suspension. Grief is paused. Instead, there is an adrenaline that carries most of us through those first days after a bereavement.

For many long-term carers, their immediate emotions will be complicated and contradictory. Loss and sadness, of course, but possibly also relief that their loved one isn't suffering anymore and they don't have to witness it. And that relief is often tinged with guilt at the realisation they might sleep a little later, not always having to think of someone else's medication, someone else's hospital appointments, presiding over their remorseless decline, watching powerless as their body fails them.

There are so many arrangements to be made: obituaries to be written, the undertakers to be appointed and the funeral service finalised. Then, there are the financial matters – the dead person's assets and responsibilities, which draws carers into a complex web of official notifications and paperwork. For widows in more traditional marriages, it can be bewildering without help. Phone calls and emails, the 'I'm sorry to say I'm ringing to tell you that our beloved father died on Wednesday ...' Will there be a burial or a cremation, where might the wake be held? So much to do. We keep ourselves occupied and busy with practical things so as not to be left alone with our grief.

Then, it's over. The visitors go back to wherever they came from and the bereaved are left with the reality of living with the empty chair at the kitchen table, the space on the other side of the bed. This is when the magnitude of the loss hits home. The bleak realisation that this – now – is how it is. That there will always – now – be an absence. All the things that you did together, the two of you, will lose their shine. If you can bring yourself to carry on doing them at all.

Some grieving carers are left completely without help – the women who gave up their jobs to care for a parent or a spouse, those with little or no family close at hand. For them, there's not only loneliness, but possibly hardship too. A significant reduction in household income, losing not only the carer's allowance, if applicable, but possibly the benefits of a joint pension as well. Too many sole carers find themselves struggling financially at precisely the moment when they most need support.

*

Loneliness is the scourge of our age. My father's paid carers would often arrive distressed by having left a client who, they knew, would not speak to another living soul until the same time the following morning. We live in unprecedented times, where technology can link us to others in any corner of the globe. But for older people, whose eyesight may be failing or whose hearing aids are not compatible with mobile phones or who find the technology too bewildering, it is easy to become isolated.

In Japan, adult adoption is a centuries' old tradition, originally developed as a mechanism for families to extend their family name, estate and ancestry without a reliance on bloodlines. In the UK, successive governments and local authorities have tried, with varying degrees of success, to set up 'adopt a granny' schemes, or foster links between local care homes and schools.

The charity helpline Silverline was launched by Esther Rantzen in 2012, partly in reaction to her own experiences of being widowed at the age of seventy-one and finding herself living alone. Working now in partnership with Age UK, Silverline offers free confidential advice to any older person who needs it – and there is a very great need. Of the estimated 11.4 million people over the age of sixty-five in the UK, some 3.5 million of them live alone. Over the age of seventy-five, there are still 2 million single-person households, of whom 1.5 million are women. Many, of course, are happy and healthy, supported by family and friends. But others are alone and lonely, inspiring Britain's most-loved centenarian – Captain Sir Tom Moore – to launch a podcast in October 2020 to combat isolation, becoming the oldest podcast host in the UK in the process and, as the second national lockdown started, to begin walking again – 'Walk with Tom' – to raise funds for those who are isolated.

My mother met my father when she was nineteen. They had been together for sixty years. Now, they were not.

My sisters and I were worried that Ma might decide that it simply wasn't worth the effort to adjust to life without him. She was nearly eighty and had lived almost her entire adulthood life in his company. We feared she might lose spirit, or be unable to recover from the last few months of such exhaustion. Grieving is a process, the books tell us so. It can't be hurried. It follows its own rules and cadence. The heart takes its time to come back to life. But we brought her little presents to lighten the days: my youngest sister was queen of the liquorice allsorts and the daffodils, my middle sister would talk about her own grandsons and Ma's recipe for her legendary 'orange chicken'.

But, though grieving and a little shell-shocked, she turned out to be more resilient and determined than any of us expected. She did want to find her way forward, and though she missed him terribly, she wasn't frightened of life on her own. Unlike many carers, she had not withdrawn from the world during my father's decline. His horizons had gradually shrunk as his Parkinson's symptoms became more difficult to manage, but Ma had continued to be out and about in so far as she could.

One of the most bolstering things for her – for us all – was the great affection people felt for my father. It seemed every post would bring another batch of cards. Hundreds and hundreds of them, the cards and letters kept coming. Most were from extended family, friends and known colleagues. But others came from virtual strangers, speaking of my father's kindness to them in a time of need or of how he had done something – sometimes fifty years in the past or more – that had made a difference to their lives. The words 'honourable' and 'kind' came up time and again, though it was the word 'gentleman' that appeared most.

It was a great comfort. Talking about him gave Ma a way to remember the man he'd been before the illness took hold and to celebrate everything he'd achieved during his life. To feel proud of him. No longer someone to be cared for, someone who was suffering, in her memory my father could be himself again. She didn't want to move on too quickly, but it was a relief to be able to allow the recent past – the past of illness and distress and hospitals – to fade and their sixty years of life together to come to the fore. The condolence cards and the photograph albums, often brought down from the shelf, gave her a way to keep the spirit of him alive. And they helped her adjust to being a widow rather than a wife.

After someone has died, the 'firsts' are the worst – the first anniversary, the first Christmas. Everyone understands this. They creep up on us, these familiar landmarks. We can all be hit with an odd feeling of disloyalty, as if it's wrong to be carrying on without them. We feel guilty if, for a moment like Orpheus, we forget their unique expressions, their smile, their laugh, the way they took their tea. The scent on a coat left abandoned on the back of the door. The clouds lift and you forget to be sad. Then you remember, and feel guilty. Holding on to the pain of their loss is a way of holding on to them.

My father's own birthday and my parents' wedding anniversary in May had been swallowed up in the time between his death and the funeral. Now it was September, the month – in Elizabeth von Arnim's words – 'of quiet days, crimson creepers, and blackberries'. My mother's eightieth birthday was fast approaching on the fifteenth and she was dreading it.

She insisted she didn't want anything much, but my sisters, my daughter and I did manage to whisk her off for a day in a spa. Afterwards, when we were all primped and shining, we had supper out. But still, it was the first time in sixty years that there hadn't been a birthday card propped up on the breakfast table addressed in my father's appalling handwriting, the first time without a parcel from him to open. And no matter how many gifts we bought, or how many outings were arranged to favourite places, nothing would ever make up for that absence.

No one knows what really goes on inside another marriage or relationship, even when you live at the closest quarters. There's no doubt that there were frustrations and impatience, days of despair and irritation, moments when it all seemed too much or too unfair, that powerlessness again. There were disappointments, and sadnesses, and things that didn't work out. Days of love and days of pity for the way of things. Children tend to romanticise their parents, perhaps. But, all the same, I can't shake the haunting melody of Jacques Brel's 'La Chanson des Vieux Amants' – 'The Old Lovers' – from my head, as he swears to his beloved how, from first light to the close of day, he will always love her.

10

North of Eighty

I'VE ALWAYS LOVED CHRISTMAS. Everything about it. I love going to the garden centre to choose a Nordmann fir, its needles shimmering somewhere between green and blue and heavy with the scent of pine. I love the pleasure of hunting for the perfect present.

When my sisters and I were little, we had advent calendars with chocolates for each day of the month. We'd watch my father climb up the stepladder into the loft and bring down the cardboard boxes containing last year's tinsel and baubles. Ma hung all the Christmas cards around the house on lengths of red cotton. With our hearts in our mouths, we'd wait as the plug was switched on to see if the tree lights were still working.

It's not true for everyone of course, but if you have happy memories of Christmases past, you are likely to replicate them or attempt to: a fixed sequence of events, jokes that become shabbier every year with retelling, mince pies that nobody wants. This is how family history and traditions are made and it's these memories that can sustain you in the dark times, during the grieving times.

Was Christmas different that first year? Were the colours less bright, the smiles more reserved, the traditional joys of the season overshadowed by the fact my father was no longer with us? In all honesty, I can't remember. It's like trying to put a treasured old jigsaw puzzle back together only to discover that several of the key pieces in the middle are missing.

For any carer, the sudden liberation from tasks and concerns that have given structure to one's daily life for years can feel like the scaffolding falling down around your ears.

Many of the carers I spoke to told me of how, after the first weeks of 'freedom', they found it increasingly difficult to know what to do with their time. Of feeling purposeless. Others talked of lacking the will to pick up hobbies they'd let slide or reconnecting with friends whom they'd cancelled once too often. Older carers, particularly widows and widowers, mentioned feeling they'd somehow got out of step with the outside world. Some end up confining their lives even further, having shopping delivered, preferring to remain at home with their books, the radio or the television for company. The world just seems too noisy, too chaotic.

In the Covid-19 lockdowns of 2020–21, people across the country – across the whole world – experienced this kind of confinement. Overnight, everyone learned what it was like not to be able to go out when they wanted. How it felt not to be able to see friends or family. How it felt to be hyper vigilant of their own health for fear of inadvertently introducing illness into a household where someone was vulnerable.

'Unpaid carers are the pillars of our health and social care systems,' wrote Helen Walker, the chief executive of Carers UK in June 2020, 'yet many say they feel invisible and ignored.'

Now, everybody had a better understanding of what it meant to be a carer. Suddenly, carers' work was being applauded and seen. For some of us caring at home, rather than being at the mercy of a system under huge strain, there was almost an odd sense of relief about lockdown at first. We were no longer the outsiders, the ones making excuses for not being able to attend some evening meeting or for having to leave early.

But for most who had a watching brief for older relatives who lived elsewhere, it was devastating. The worry about what would happen if their mother or father fell or didn't have enough food in the house. Not being able to explain to those suffering with dementia or Alzheimer's. Anxiety became constant. Not being able to visit, not being able to hug or speak properly except through glass. For those in care homes, the situation was even more distressing. More than 14,000 residents died in care homes in the UK during the first six months of Covid-19, a figure that was kept artificially low by poor reporting and accounting.

The cruelty and lack of respect was disgraceful. In Frances Harper's words, as true today as in 1866:

We are all bound up together in one bundle of humanity, and society cannot trample on the weakest and feeblest of its members without receiving the curse in its own soul.

With essential human contact denied during the first – and successive – national lockdowns, so many of the things that give an older person's life meaning were taken away from them without negotiation. The effect on people's mental health was catastrophic. The final tally, of those who should not have died within the care system, will be heartbreaking. So very many friends spoke of the desperation they felt at not being able to comfort those they loved, or explain to them what was happening.

Though Rosie has lived with us for more than twenty years, she has remained on friendly terms with her third husband, who is in a care home in Bognor. They had known each other from the 1930s in Apuldram and, as she says, 'there's hardly anyone else left'. Before Covid, she would visit every other week. Since March 2020, she's not been able to see him at all. In his early nineties, with failing sight and failed hearing, his comprehension is limited. But Rosie remains troubled by the idea that he might think she's abandoned him.

In October 2020, as the UK entered a period of regional lockdowns and then the second national lockdown, the Care Quality Commission insisted the long-overdue reform of the care system 'needs to happen now – not at some point in the future', and that ministers' failure to act was turning inequalities in the health sector – not least of all in provision for disabled young people and black communities, and people of colour who were being disproportionately affected by Covid – from 'faultlines into chasms'.

Following the release of 'Caring Behind Closed Doors' – reporting that many carers did not think they could survive the winter without help – Carers UK launched a campaign to raise the carers' allowance, and exhorting people to write to their local MPs demanding that the well-being and practical needs of carers were taken seriously. As of March 2021, these issues remain unresolved.

In those first months after my father's death in 2011, I missed him all the time but without ever wishing he was still with us.

The challenges of physical decline had become too burdensome to him, too distressing for him and for my mother. He wanted dignity and agency, both of which became less and less possible. He had been ready to go. All the same, I often found myself looking up to the sky and talking to him. Little things that I thought he'd like to know, or would amuse him, or make him proud. Letting him know we were looking after Ma. The usual ebbs and flows of a life.

In the last six months of his life, I'd stopped travelling for work, just in case something happened while I was away. I had an idea for a new historical adventure series, but I was creatively worn out and it would have required research that would take me out of the country. (I didn't know it then, but it wouldn't be until 2016 that the clouds would lift and I fell back in love with this project.) Greg was always there, my sisters were there, but I still wanted to stay close to home, to be on hand if need be.

All the same, I didn't want to not write. So, for the first time since my earliest attempts at fiction, I turned to the immediate world outside my window.

I do most of the 'writing' of a first draft in my head, while walking. I always felt particularly close to my father in our shared Sussex landscape, the county celebrated by William Blake and John Marsh and, of course, Kipling, so I wrote a series of short, winter stories. A few were inspired by Cathar and Breton folklore, but the majority were based on the mythology and traditions of the landscape through which I walked and had, so many years before, walked with my father.

Climbing the steep chalk-and-flint path up to the Iron Age Trundle above West Dean and into Kingley Vale, the oldest yew forest in Europe. By legend, the oldest of the trees – a circle in the green heart of the woods – sprang up centuries ago where the Saxon defenders of the Sussex Weald died protecting their land against the Viking invaders. Around them, year on year, the forest spread. Dark trunks, twisted roots, red sap, their branches dabbling at the earth like skeletal fingers. Lichen, moss, the wet living soil. A habitat for butterflies and birds, fallow deer and hare.

The forest is animate, careless of human emotions, ever changing and never changing. When I journeyed along those wine-coloured pathways, in the presence of these magnificent trees, I was reminded of how very short a human lifespan is. How the truth of our lived and imagined experiences lies in the land itself. There, I felt connected profoundly to a past that is enduring and true. I was reassured that our stories go on.

It is peaceful at the heart of the woods.

These days when I'm walking, I prefer to walk alone. Thinking, keeping sane, trying to manage my stress and unwelcome anxieties. But even if I'd invited her, my mother wouldn't have wanted to come. She could have managed, but striding across the countryside in wellington boots was never her thing.

Ma didn't need care in the same way that my father had. She managed all her own medication and hospital appointments, though one of us would often drop her off or pick her up. But, having lived with someone for nearly sixty years, she did need companionship. She and Granny Rosie were chalk and cheese, very different sorts of women with diametrically opposed life experiences of marriage and partnership. Yet, they soon fell into a pattern.

Every morning, Ma would drive early to the corner shop to get the papers, then would come into our kitchen for coffee where she and Rosie would scrap and scrabble over the crossword – both of them avid fans, though owing allegiance to different newspapers, the *Telegraph* and the *Daily Express* respectively. I could often hear the negotiations from my study.

Only a year apart in age, sometimes they compared their experiences of the war. Whereas Ma had been evacuated from Woolwich to Wales, then to Yorkshire, Rosie had remained at home with her family in Apuldram. Because London was still suffering from the Blitz, the Chi grammar girls had had to share their premises with evacuees from a girls' school in Croydon. They had the mornings, the visitors the afternoons.

They had both been teachers too, though, again, their experiences were very different. Ma had worked with secondary or college students, teaching business studies and economics. Rosie started with infants, then juniors and finally, at the end of her career, working as a senior teacher at the local school for children with severe physical and learning disabilities.

Of all her jobs, Rosie most often reminisced about her time at Fordwater special school. Even many years after retiring, whenever she walked through Chichester, odds were that a former parent would rush up to greet her, a smile wide with gratitude. 'You haven't changed a bit, Mrs Turner. I'd know you anywhere.' Rosie rarely remembers a parent's face or name, but she never forgets the pupils themselves. She looked beyond the disability and took everyone as she finds them.

She still does.

Although they both had their grumbles – and had 'views' on one another's driving – they would sometimes go for a midweek 'ladies' lunch' at our local pub. They were always given the same table in the corner. Because of the warfarin, Ma felt the cold keenly, so they gave her a chair with its back to the radiator and brought her hot elderflower cordial in a glass, to keep Rosie company with her G&T. (Ma was teetotal – she'd never drunk alcohol.) All through lunch they would 'watch the room' for the comings and goings. Then, at the end of the meal, Ma would twist the gold wrappers of the mint chocolates into perfect, tiny goblets and bring them home.

The importance of older people having company of their own age, even if they have little else in common, is often underestimated. But we all understand what a relief it can be to have someone who simply knows and remembers the world that you once knew. Someone who has a similar frame of reference. Besides, Greg and I had met as teenagers – he was at the boys' comp next door to the girls' school – so Ma and Rosie had known each other a long time.

The first anniversary of my father's death in May 2012 was difficult. But a few days later, my mother came with Greg, Felix and me to see Martha's art degree final show in Brighton and loved it.

Many carers, and those with older parents, talk about the importance of grandchildren. How sometimes a parent can rejoice and re-engage with the world better through that next generation down and can be lifted by their youth, their enthusiasm, that sense of being at the beginning of their lives. Visits or time spent with a granddaughter or grandson can be the tonic that's needed. The grandchildren of a friend, whose husband had developed early-onset Alzheimer's, recorded a film for him with photographs of her, her brother and sister, so their father could keep their faces clear in his mind. It was one of the things that kept him going when none of them could be with him during the Covid lockdowns. My mother loved going to Weald & Downland Living Museum with my youngest sister and her girls, she loved seeing my middle sister with her own grandchildren.

I wish I'd asked Ma more about how hard she was finding it to look forward rather than backwards. But, at the time, I think I was grateful that she seemed happy. As the months passed, she continued to re-establish her old life – or reconfigure a new version of it step by step. Her diary was filling up. She had her heart issues and COPD, but her health was otherwise not too bad. She joined a local choir and I can remember how I cried when I saw her up on that stage for the first time singing her socks off with her new friends. This wasn't something she had done when my father was alive, but something completely new.

Something for just her.

After the triumph of the choir, Rosie persuaded Ma to join her entertainment troupe, the Old Timers. So called, as Rosie always says, 'not because we were old' – though the average age was somewhere north of eighty – but, rather, because 'we played the old-time songs'.

When we moved back to Sussex from London in 1998, Greg, Martha, Felix and I had gone to our first Old Timers' performance to support Granny Rosie. Although the troupe's *raison d'être* was to take lively entertainment year-round to care homes, hospitals, hospices and day centres – raising money for the local minibus fund in the process – they gave an annual gala for the public in the spring. The village hall was packed. A local crowd of family and friends, tea from an urn and warm white wine, raffle tickets and orange squash, bourbon biscuits in plastic wrappers.

Rosie is a brilliant entertainer: funny, unscripted, in her words 'a real one-off'. She gave a running commentary from her piano, peppered with jokes about the performers being 'on her deaf side' and having no idea what key she was supposed to be in. Or what the next song might be. Everyone on the stage was significantly past retirement age and happy to throw themselves enthusiastically into anything. No one minded if people forgot the words, or made an entrance at the wrong time.

A lady in her nineties with reduced sight was walked to the front of the stage to sing 'Itsy Bitsy Teenie Weenie Yellow Polka Dot Bikini', wearing her costume over the top of her everyday clothes. She brought the house down. There was an Abba medley and a rollicking version of 'When Father Papered the Parlour', a few saucy numbers from the 1940s with winks and nudges, and a distinguished-looking gentleman in a blonde wig and dirndl checked skirt sang 'High on a Hill was a Lonely Goatherd'.

During the interval, the raffle.

Knowing Granny Rosie doesn't like wine, someone rustled up a gin and tonic and placed it within reach on the edge of the stage. Finally, every one of the thirty raffle prizes had been claimed – including a tin of corned beef – and the audience was back in their seats, ready for the second half to begin. One of the performers, a man dressed as an elf, turned the heavy crank handle and the red curtain jerked back. Rosie's 'restorative' was launched into the audience.

This was not the kind of environment I would ever have imagined my mother in. Her love of theatre had been, until now, on the auditorium side of the footlights. But, eighteen months after my father's death, as the newest recruit to the Old Timers, Ma throws herself into it. She brings a touch of glamour and has a killer pair of legs in fishnet tights. When she recites Roald Dahl's 'Red Riding Hood' and pulls the pistol from her knickers to shoot the wolf dead, she does it with the confidence of a variety performer. Her career and her recent years of caring for my father have not prepared her for this, but she's wonderful.

11

Food, Glorious Food

MY MOTHER WAS A GOOD COOK, though she didn't particularly enjoy cooking.

When we were children, we sat down to supper together at six o'clock every weekday evening, once my father was back from the office. Casseroles and fish pies, pork chops and mashed potato, chicken in white sauce. For pudding, apple pie and custard or, my father's favourite, jam roly-poly. Even when I went off fish at the age of about eight, and stopped eating meat at the age of ten, Ma took it in her stride. I had the roast without the meat, the toad-in-the-hole without the sausages.

Being the main cook in a family is a tie, an obligation. It's also boring, to be forever thinking about meals if it's not your bag. One of the things Ma said she enjoyed, once all three of us girls were old enough to fend for ourselves, was not having to think so much about food shopping and catering. Cooking a lamb roast on a Sunday, for special occasions and favourite meals, that was all fine. But it didn't occupy some of her thoughts for some of every day. I feel the same. Left to my own devices, I'd survive on Marmite toast and baked potatoes. The occasional grape. There are other things I'd rather be doing.

Though there were celebrity chefs in the 1960s and 70s, food wasn't the obsession it is now. Talking about food, travelling to 'experience' food, photographing, imagining, rejecting, disliking, dreaming, constructing rather than simply 'cooking'. In the first two decades of the twenty-first century it's become a major source of entertainment.

Much of our social and working lives revolve around food too, another ordinary communal activity that was suspended during the pandemic. The ritual of eating with someone else, or cooking for someone else, can be an act of affection, or charity, or courtship or love. From evenings spent in a special restaurant to the daily sandwich bought to punctuate the working day, from biscuits in the staffroom to cake in the office on someone's birthday, we communicate with one another through the providing and sharing of food.

Hand in glove with this, we are bombarded all the time with messages about healthy eating, about what a balanced diet looks like (though this so often ignores the differences between women and men, between different ethnicities, between different cultures, different ages). Sometimes the simple pleasure of just choosing what you fancy is stripped away. And this complex, even dysfunctional relationship with food, ignores the fact that many people in the world still do not have enough to eat, that in the UK, one of the world's richest countries, there are now food banks in every town.

For carers, food can be a battlefield and the constant dialogue about it can be counterproductive.

Many older people, whether they are living comfortably alone or need some measure of support, might be struggling to summon up any real interest in food – perhaps their digestion is working overtime, perhaps they no longer notice they are hungry and believe that their tiredness is a symptom of old age not lack of fuel.

It's common for older people to lose their appetites. They might be taking medication that destroys their taste buds. Issues with dentures might mean they can no longer cope with the foods that gave them pleasure – too crunchy, too sticky, too spicy, too fiddly, contraindicated with essential medication. Like my father, the physical act of eating might have become burdensome.

Many carers worry that the person they're caring for is eating too little, or eating too little of the 'right' thing. Of course, a balanced diet with plenty of fruit and veg is excellent, but the last thing any elderly woman or man wants to be told is what's good or bad for them or what they 'ought' to have. Doctor's orders, maybe, but at this stage in life, the habit of sensible, healthy eating maybe matters less than getting anything eaten at all.

There might be the indignity of no longer being able to feed oneself, or feeling watched or observed, so that eating becomes an act of endurance rather than of pleasure. Nutrition and calories matter, because that's the most reliable way to make sure someone has the strength and power to fight an infection. But if you have lost your appetite, being coaxed to eat against your wishes as if you are a child will feel like yet a further loss of independence. All the same, for carers, it is a constant source of worry. It's easy to become fixated on how little (or too much of the wrong thing) the person for whom you're caring is eating. When I'm grumbling at Rosie when she hasn't wanted anything more than a single piece of toast for days, she'll often come back at me: 'Yes, Mum!' and I'll apologise for being a pain.

It's a disquieting role reversal.

Susie Orbach said that 'fat is a feminist issue', and it's as true in 2021 as it was in 1978 when her polemic was first published. Depending on a woman's own sense of herself, how comfortable she feels within her own skin, with her own size and fitness, this area can become even more complicated. Women and girls (and increasingly boys and men too) are bombarded constantly about body image, about appearance, bullied for their weight and their shape and their looks. Many women become carers around the same time as they are going through the menopause, when our hormones and emotions are all over the shop. For those who are struggling to maintain a positive self-image, looking after someone who seems to be fading away before your eyes will be additionally challenging.

Hunger is the sensible reason for eating, yet we all use food to pass the time or to give ourselves a 'treat'. For carers, this sense of being confined inside and needing to help the hours pass often means taking refuge in the biscuit jar, too many cups of coffee, the odd KitKat to keep the energy levels up in the middle of a long afternoon, a packet of peanuts. (My particular poison is Mini Cheddars.) Since many carers struggle with self-esteem, this spiral of snacking and eating too much of the 'wrong' food, followed by regret, is not helpful and can add to a sense of failure.

Of course, ensuring that the person you're caring for is eating properly is one of the few concrete things a carer can do to make a difference. There's no cure for old age. There's no way of reversing the effects of a life-limiting illness. And if eating together equals companionship, then the failure to tempt someone to eat equals rejection, bringing in its wake frustration, impatience, resentment. It's a skip and a jump to every mealtime becoming a skirmish, with both sides left disappointed and worn out. Again, many parents know the danger of allowing mealtimes to become emotional rather than practical. There's a peculiar kind of misery when you prepare food that no one wants, or will not or cannot eat.

Old habits die hard. And many older people become diabetic, so following an appropriate diet as recommended by the doctor is essential. But if we try to let go of the 'ought to have' and instead try to embrace 'what do you fancy?', the path can be, if not frictionless, then certainly easier.

Does it matter if your 90-year-old father only wants to eat a choc ice today? Or your 85-year-old mother only wants to snack on Mint Matchmakers? It's better than nothing.

What's essential is to find things that appeal, that tempt, that are simple to eat and can play a part in maintaining appetite. And, though it can be hard work, structured mealtimes are a big help. They are social and remind of easier times when food was enjoyable, not another burden. Some older people, especially those with neurological deficits, will struggle to remember if they've eaten or cope with questions about what they might want to eat. Women in particular have often spent a lifetime not asking for anything, training themselves to be modest in their requirements. Sometimes, just putting something tasty down on the table might do the trick.

My mother had been through all of this with my father.

Now, liberated from the daily responsibility of caring for someone else, she was free to eat what she liked, and when she liked. A tray on her knees in front of the television, if she fancied, with tomatoes on toast, or a fried egg, a prawn sandwich. She loved a proper Sunday lunch at my youngest sister's house that she hadn't had to cook, or a bowl of soup with friends, or kitchen suppers with us on a free-for-all Saturday night. But, mostly, she turned her back on big meals, hot and sloppy cooking, and ate in the way she would have done if she hadn't had a family to look after. If she wanted to eat peanut butter from the jar with a spoon, then why not ...?

In 2013, the doctor felt she was too thin and prescribed some awful, claggy vitamin supplement drinks. She hated them. And I didn't want to nag, so pretended not to notice that the same number of bottles were sitting in the fridge at the end of the week as at the beginning. It was another important way that she was recalibrating life in her widowhood, allowing herself to choose.

12

Four Days in Belfast

MA'S CARING ROLE HAD GONE and mine was yet to come. I didn't think time was short, even though there were one or two occasions when her breathing caused her trouble or the balance of her medication got a little out of kilter.

In the 1940s, smoking was promoted as stylish, attractive and good for your nerves. The pages of golden age detective stories – Georgette Heyer, Ngaio Marsh, Josephine Tey, Patricia Wentworth – are filled with heroines smoking. They are cool, collected and determined young women. The fact they smoke is a definition of character, not an unnecessary piece of description.

My mother started smoking when she started working, and had never stopped. Her mother was a smoker – my sisters and I would watch with horrified pleasure as Granny's ash got longer and longer, taking bets on when it would fall. My father used to smoke. My husband and my sisters, too. I'd been a Silk Cut girl. In my early twenties, working as a secretary in a publishing company in London, smoking by the photocopier made the time pass more quickly. Then, in my mid-twenties, I caught the flu. Proper flu that had me off work and in bed for three weeks. When I recovered, I went into a tobacconist on the Tottenham Court Road, near to the office, and reached for the familiar white-and-purple packet and a box of matches. I always loved the sound of the scratch, then the hiss, the flare. I lit up, ready to be myself again, and hated it. The rasp in the back of the throat, the hollow taste of ash in my mouth, the smell of Soho pubs where women were not welcome.

I tried again, and again – it was part of who I was – but in the end I had to accept I was no longer a smoker.

I was incredibly lucky that the habit rejected me, rather than my having to fight to escape its poisonous arms. But I did feel a little bit less me, for a while, a little less interesting – stupid, I know.

Smoking was part of who Ma was too. Nowadays, smoking is transgressive rather than normal. It speaks of a refusal to follow the trend, a refusal to be dictated to. She stayed loyal to Embassy, never moving on to the now standard 'king size', standing at her kitchen window looking out over the flowerbeds she'd planted. Embassy are short, two drags and a spit, and truthfully, I think it was more about the feel of holding the cigarette than smoking it.

My sisters and I nagged her to stop, which pissed her off and made us feel we were somehow failing in our duty. Ma didn't want us to treat her like a child though. She knew what damage smoking could do – and had done – and decided it was worth the risk. But, of course, each winter, there was always the threat of a slight cold becoming a chest infection. Visits to the COPD clinic. A few times, we needed to call an ambulance in the middle of the night. Once or twice, they kept her in hospital. Other times, the wonderful paramedics would serve up a little oxygen, like providing a cup of tea, and wait until all was well.

These incidents became a little more common. I began to go to bed with my phone on the floor next to me once again. And often, wakeful in the night, I'd see the light go on in Ma's kitchen at three in the morning and know she was also up, doing the crossword. I'd wait until it snapped off, and all was dark, before going back to my own bed too.

Aside from her COPD, Ma was otherwise well. She had a standing prescription for antibiotics to make sure that any potential chest infection was knocked on the head before it had a chance to take hold. But she still had plenty of enthusiasm for life.

Certain memories stick out. Going up to London with her and her two best friends, also in their eighties, to see the theatre show Felix was appearing in. Again, many older people will find the energy for outings or special occasions involving grandchildren. They want to be fully present in their lives, if they can. Ma was broad-minded, free-thinking, but she and 'the girls' were slightly startled by the language and the storyline of *The Book of Mormon*.

So much so that she launched herself at the wrong blond boy at the stage door afterwards to congratulate him. The right granny, the wrong Mormon ...

I remember, too, receiving an exciting piece of news and rushing in with the letter to Ma's kitchen to tell her. Remember her delight, then her tears that my father wasn't here to see it, knowing he would have been so proud. It was one of those tiny reminders that, however fine everything seemed on the surface, she missed him and missed having someone to share things with. I know it was those quiet moments at home, sitting alone in her kitchen in the night or watching a television programme they'd both liked on her own, that were the loneliest.

In August 2014, we decided on a family girls' trip to Belfast – me, Ma, Granny Rosie and Martha. Neither of the mums had ever been to Northern Ireland and everyone needed a change of scene before the winter set in.

Rosie was walking with a stick, so we needed to allow plenty of time for getting through the airport, and Martha and I worked out how we could carry the baggage between us. There were several last-minute checks for medication, for inhalers, for any of the essential essentials that two ladies in their eighties away from home might need.

My mother used to love travelling, but this was the first time she had been on a plane since the flight in 2004 when my father became ill. Airports are noisy places, frantic and unforgiving. Loud. Rosie wears a hearing aid and is none too quick on her pins and Ma can get breathless if she has to rush or walk too fast. I didn't want either of them to feel under pressure.

But as we take off from Gatwick, I catch a glance at her face, and she is exhilarated. This is a remembrance of freer times, a literal letting-go of the past ten years, and it's brilliant. I squeeze my daughter's hand, and she understands.

We hit the shops, we visit the Giant's Causeway in County Antrim – the magnificent 40,000 interlocking basalt columns caused by a volcanic eruption – and it's every bit as awe-inspiring as we'd hoped. An ancient landscape of grey stone, green headland and wide blue skies. For both Rosie and my mother, it's been a lifelong ambition to stand and stare. In the years ahead, for Rosie and me, the effort needed to cope with travel will become too much to make it worth the candle. So my advice is that while it's still possible to help someone to tick things off on their bucket list late into their lives, then do it if you can. It's important that healthy older people are supported and not made to feel that they're no longer allowed to aim for things or dream or have new experiences.

We have the sweetest photograph of the mums together in their cagoules – Ma's a livid leaf green, Rosie's a more sensible navy blue – sitting on a bench. Their hair buffeted by the wind, they are each holding a pair of knitted woollen birds in their hands (Granny Rosie's latest project for the children's hospice shop), pulling faces and laughing.

On the way back to our hotel, we stop at the Bushmills Distillery. My father is much in our minds – he loved whiskey. I'm the designated driver and, in any case, I can't bear spirits, my mother is teetotal, Martha has a sip and wrinkles her nose, so Granny Rosie ends up with all four of the post-tour samples of single malt and does her best.

Later, we enjoy a farewell dinner in the hotel overlooking the shipyard where the *Titanic* was built. We raise a toast to what we pledge will be the first of many excursions. As the evening marches on, our suggestions of where we might go next become more and more ambitious until we are circling the globe. Like Jules Verne and Freya Stark or Gertrude Bell, we will be adventurers. Shaking the dust off our tired old heels and cutting free – irresponsible, footloose, defying expectations in search of new experiences. Like Agatha Christie, we will embrace a wild and unexpected life:

I like living. I have sometimes been wildly, despairingly, acutely miserable, racked with sorrow; but through it all I still know quite certainly that just to be alive is a grand thing.

We don't really mean it of course, but it was an expression of there being things for us all to look forward to. Of pleasure in one another's company and planning for the future.

We give back the hire car, climb onto the plane, and fly home with our batteries recharged. Martha has photographs of our road trip made up into two albums, one for Rosie and one for Ma, for Christmas. A memento of our four days in Belfast.

Two weeks later, her spirits revived, Ma books herself onto a river cruise on the Rhine with an old friend. Job done, I thought. This is her new normal.

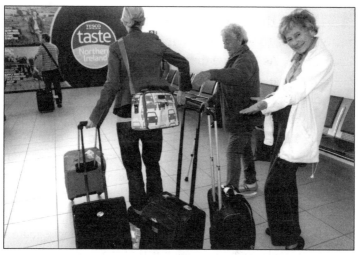

Me, Granny Rosie and Ma, Belfast Airport, August 2014

13

The Shortest Day

LOOKING BACK, DID I MISS the signs, or not want to see them for what they were? Should I have known? In novels, in plays, in films, the music tells us how to recognise a moment of significance or that a storm is approaching. That, contrary to all appearances, we are in the home straight.

It's one of the most common regrets among carers – that the moment when the crisis comes looks so precisely like all the other moments of crisis that you don't realise it is something different until it's too late.

In September 2014, I launched my latest novel to a home crowd in Chichester. Ma, splendid in cream jacket and black trousers, heckled happily from the audience, contradicting my rather saccharine accounts of my childhood and love for the Marshes. She was witty, proud and delighted to see Fishbourne put on the page.

All the same, I was rather out of sorts. Not nervous so

much as jittery. As if I was anticipating trouble. Although I'd enjoyed writing the novel, the usual frills and bells around publication had given me little pleasure. For the first time, going out and about to bookshops and events felt like work, not fun.

My reading habits changed, too. Most of my to-be-read pile is fiction, classics past and present, pretty much anything. If I went to London, I'd nip into the WH Smith at Victoria Station for a new paperback novel to keep me company on the way home. And even though my reading for research was almost all non-fiction – plenty of biography and theology, military history, books about medieval Christianity and warfare, women in the Resistance or World War II campaigns – the perfect Sunday afternoon would be a glass of wine, curled up and reading a story by the fire.

This adjustment from fiction to non-fiction happened slowly, unobserved. Unremarked. Finding my hands going to the 'wrong' shelves in a bookshop: Ann Patchett reflecting on her marriage and Atul Gawande's *Being Mortal*. I wasn't seeking guidance – at least, not consciously – but Gawande's book was a catalyst to thought, to contemplation, to analysing why the world we are living in fails to deliver dignity, power, choice and humanity to so many at the end of their lives. Henry Marsh's *Do No Harm*, Robert McCrum's searingly honest *My Year Off* and Helen McDonald's *H is for Hawk* – personal books all, though with some broader underlying truth. Life-writing capturing a moment or an emotion, stories from the real world.

It felt odd to be turning my back on fiction, but intriguing all the same – like finding oneself in an unexpected conversation at a party. A sense of eavesdropping on someone else's thinking aloud, other writers saying listen to me.

Books about how to die and how to die well.

In November, my mother goes on her river cruise. Her wallet is stolen, but she remains robust and furious and I'm amazed at how she takes it in her stride.

In December, with Christmas fast approaching, I have to go abroad for research. My husband comes too, so my youngest sister holds the fort at home, keeping an eye on Rosie as well as Ma. She's been having problems with her teeth and my sister is sorting out all of the appointments and treatment for her. But I'm distracted, not really able to concentrate and ring home every day.

Then we're back and straight into one last crazy busy week up and down to London – meeting after meeting, which is unusual. I feel on edge, as if I'm not properly paying attention to anything. In Stevie Smith's famous words, 'not waving but drowning'. I'm impatient and short-tempered, worn out by the competing demands on my time. When I land back in Chichester, Ma is clearly very tired and breathless, though still going out and about: a visit to the dentist, lunch with her 'girls'. She's well enough to perform onstage, well enough to go last-minute shopping with my youngest sister, well enough to write all her Christmas cards.

I put them in the post. So many friends, from all parts of her life.

On the Friday, she is having trouble breathing. Fearing it's another chest infection, the doctor comes – as he has, on and off, for the previous couple of weeks, and sternly orders her to eat more, to rest and no more rushing about. We all laugh. As if Ma will sit still at Christmas – and she still hasn't made the brandy butter. Though trying to take it easy, she is full of winks and nods, enjoying all the comings and goings. Her eyes twinkle with mischievous glee at the presents she's bought for us, for her grandchildren, for her great-grandchildren.

During the night, something happens. It's never clear quite what.

Early in the morning, I call 111 and then 999. Taking no risks. The ambulance comes – quickly, discreetly. No siren or flashing blue light. After a deal of discussion – the paramedics are not sure it's necessary – it's decided that it might be sensible to go to hospital. Better safe than sorry. There's a deal of joking and gossip in the rig and Ma responds, though she is struggling to catch her breath.

Many carers know their loved ones have a fear of being taken to hospital and the papers are often full of descriptions of what happens if the system is overwhelmed and care there fails – patients lying on trolleys in corridors, older people or those who have difficulty expressing themselves, not having anything to drink or eat, the depression of the wards. In very busy cities, there can be an anonymity that turns every individual into simply a number on a form. Philip Larkin's poem 'The Building' puts into words what most people feel at that moment:

All know they are going to die.
Not yet, perhaps not here, but in the end,
And somewhere like this.

But Ma is glad to be going to the hospital. In the past, when admitted as an inpatient if her COPD breathing had become too raggedy, I'd arrive on the ward to find her brightening the atmosphere. It was a familiar place and she felt safe in the hospital, cared for, confident that her needs would be acknowledged and attended to.

At A&E, the doctors and nurses are wonderful. Efficient, compassionate, wanting to know who my mother is as a person. My sisters arrive. An Iranian doctor on secondment talks about Ma being 'rich in years' and I am grateful to her for that kindness. There are saturation tests and blood pressure, oxygen and breathing. They are doing all the usual things but, this time, nothing seems to be working.

Our experience is so far from the experience of many people at the end of life, where the apparent chaos and terror of a dash to A&E is terrifying, and bewildering and traumatic. Struggling to get answers from overworked nurses, devastating for those suffering from dementia or Alzheimer's when it might be impossible to explain. I will never stop being grateful that the hospital supported us too and did everything to treat Ma like an individual, with a long life behind her, not just another admission on a winter's afternoon close to Christmas.

As the light fades from the December sky, my husband arrives with a piece of paper. It's my mother's living will. She'd given it to Greg for safekeeping because she knew it would have been too much for us three girls to bear. Like a shadow over the future, an end point in our long, shared story that we might have tried to argue her out of.

While the consultant reads the document aloud, my sisters and I hear our mother's voice, her distinctive turn of phrase, her beautiful self telling us that she does not want to be kept artificially alive. She does not want to be incapable and cared for. She does not want be dependent on a ventilator. She wants to die as herself, being remembered as the woman she is, rather than fading away. Her words are clear and without pity, setting the terms for her leaving of life just as she set the terms for her living of it. Asking us to honour and understand her wishes.

Our mother knows what she's talking about. She cared for my father for ten years and does not want that decline for herself. It is an act of great principle, of great kindness, of great determination. It doesn't make it any easier. It's happened so quickly, so unexpectedly. I think of Emily Dickinson's words:

Because I could not stop for Death –
He kindly stopped for me.

I don't want to believe it, but my mother is dying.

The paramedics pop in on their way off duty to see how she is doing and are dismayed at the deterioration. They weren't expecting this either. Ma is no longer awake and I pray that the images imprinted on her mind are of the crisp December sunlight in her bedroom earlier, her flowers in the garden outside the window, the ordinary sounds of another day beginning, of Christmas presents wrapped and ready to go under the tree. I pray that she's thinking of turkey and cranberry sauce, not the stark neon light of A&E and worried faces.

She is slipping away, drowsy from the CO_2 that her lungs can no longer properly eradicate from her blood because they have had enough. Her heart has had enough.

The Iranian doctor finishes her shift, but does not leave. She, too, cannot quite accept that none of their measures are having any effect.

At ten o'clock that night, Ma is transferred to a ward. A ward where she's been before and the nurses remember her. They won't let us stay.

'She's a lovely lady, always so kind,' they say. 'We'll look after her,' they say. 'We'll see you in the morning.'

We don't want to leave her, but we each walk out into the cold December night, startling after hours in the artificial temperatures of the hospital. There's frost on the ground and haloes of mist hover around the streetlamps. There's an occasional car in the distance, but the whole world seems to be holding its breath.

I sit up all night, waiting for the phone to ring.

*

At 6 a.m. on Sunday 21 December, my sisters and I are called back to the hospital.

As a pale sun rises – Ma has a bed in the corner, by the window – we three sit together, keeping our beloved mother company. She does not open her eyes, but I'm sure she knows we are there.

I realise how completely unprepared I am for this. Ma never wanted to talk about that bleak side of the future – she shied away from any conversations about her wishes or what she might want when the time came – and I thought we'd have more time. Now, despite the weeks, the months, the years and years of talking and listening, I feel robbed of all those last conversations, the big statements of love and gratitude which were possible with my father because he was preparing to die. He accepted it.

My sisters feel the same, that it's all happening too fast. Despite the fact that this unexpectedly quick ending is what she wanted – what she has explicitly written down that she wants – it feels all wrong. We want to be selfish. I'm not ready to lose her. My sisters aren't ready to lose her.

My father believed he was at the beginning of a new adventure and would be reunited with those he loved. Because of his faith, he was reassured and so was I. There is no such reassurance now.

Had she been able to make the choice, I am sure Ma wouldn't have wanted to go either. But the choice she had to make was not between life or death, but between death or a living death.

And I am furious with myself. Angry. Why had I worked so hard in London during that previous week? Why wasn't I at home for every second of every day? I wish I'd never left her side because, now, here we are. I thought we had world enough and time. So many memories and reminiscences shared over the years, yet still too many words left unsaid. Too many conversations not had.

I try to find solace in the fact that the last fully conscious sight Ma had was of her own home, lying calmly surrounded by her own treasured possessions in the same bedroom where my father had died. For him, a peaceful leave-taking in May, light and colourful. For her, a bright December morning just before Christmas.

She was adored, and though I nurse a gentle hope that she is now reunited with my beloved father, it leaves our house on the corner darker and emptier and sad. Her light no longer shining below in the early mornings when I go into my study to write. She died on the shortest day of the year, when the trees were bare and the hours of light and darkness run one into the other. A day she'd always hated.

Tomorrow, the days will start to lengthen again, but she will not be here to see it.

14

In the Bleak Midwinter

DAWN IN SUSSEX. As I write this, my grief is a sharp thing. A living thing, brittle and vivid.

Overnight, the temperature has fallen. It's minus two outside, so the radio says. I can well believe it. A bleak midwinter.

The funeral is today and I can barely breathe. I've barely slept.

Grief is both universal and utterly particular. In our fifties, we enter an age where such stories are commonplace and, although each loss is personal, we hear our experiences echoed in those of our friends and extended families, in literature, painting, theatre, songs of death and remembrance, human emotions that repeat over generations, decades, centuries.

There's the memorable line in a Dylan Thomas poem, that 'After the first death, there is no other'. Though I admit it's a wilful misreading of his words, I'm furious about what a lie this is. My father's death was devastating, but the world kept turning. The death of my mother has done for me.

It still seems impossible that Ma is no longer alive. The sense of unreality began the day after she died. When I began the heartbreaking business of ringing people to tell them what had happened, some of them argued with me. They thought there must be some mistake. After all, hadn't they, that very morning, just received a Christmas card from her in the post?

Not a day goes past when I don't cry. The slightest anything sets me off. A blackbird is singing – we've chosen 'Morning Has Broken', one of her favourites, as the first hymn for her service, because she so loved the arrival of spring. This year she won't be here. The Christmas presents, including Martha's book of photographs from our Belfast trip, remain untouched under the tree. The front door to the annexe is closed and I'll never hear her key in the lock again.

I've been going into her kitchen a lot to stand in the cooling and musty air, looking out of her window on the view she loved so much. The ashtray with her lighter and packet of Embassy is still on the sill and my heart cracks a little more. The heathers she planted are holding their own, despite the frost. The dwarf roses in painted blue pots await warmer days.

The days blur.

Time is elastic, moving fast and slow. I feel almost ill all of the time. Stiff, like having a low-level flu, a blocked nose. My husband feels this too. I have nosebleeds and stomach cramps, now and then the sensation of being unable to breathe. I tell myself this is normal everyday grief, that I'm just feeling 'under the weather'.

There has been so much to do, hampered of course by the fact it was Christmas. Every day, more letters. So many letters – each one a testament to how much Ma had touched the lives of others – and I am crushed that she is not here to see how much she meant to people.

Then there is the complete disassembling of the paraphernalia and bureaucracy of a long life well lived. When my father died, there was no dismantling of hearth and home. Everything that had been theirs simply became hers. Now, my sisters and I have to decide what to sell and what to keep, what can be done with clothes or jewellery no one needs, her hats for going to the races, whose walls will make space for their paintings.

My father's walking sticks now live in a corner of my study. My mother's dressing gown, though I wouldn't dream of wearing it, hangs on a hook in our bathroom.

With my mother's death, I realised that I had never properly grieved for the loss of my father. It was so much more important to support her, to keep her going, to care for her than to give in to my own misery. Looking after her, with my husband's help and my sisters too, focused my attention away from what I was feeling. While she was alive there was still, in Henry Scott Holland's phrase, 'absolute continuity'. I didn't feel separated from who I was, from my childhood and past life, because Ma was still here. There's a hierarchy in mourning, as in everything else. Now, I'm an orphan. It's all on us. My sisters and I are the older generation. There is no one left above us.

In the three years since my father passed on – I still use this euphemism because it is what his faith allowed him to believe – I'd felt he was still with me. I've talked to him most days, inconsequential little conversations, but comforting. Now that Ma has died, he has gone too. I'd like to think it's because he has her now. That they are together, so he no longer needs to stay. But, actually, I feel doubly bereft. She has died and he, who had lingered, is now out of reach too. His calm presence no longer keeps me company on my walks on the Marshes or the Downs.

The origin of the word bereaved comes from the Old English word *berēafian*, meaning to seize, to deprive of, or to rob. Compared to many people I have been extraordinarily lucky to have both of my parents, as themselves, not lost to a fog of dementia or Alzheimer's, well into their eighties, but I still feel robbed. There is something about being an orphan, the sudden severing from your childhood. There is no longer anyone who can fill in the blanks of memories and stories, the person who provided the framework of all the days of your lived life.

I feel abandoned.

Two days ago, it was my middle sister's fiftieth birthday. It rained and rained and rained, it was the most depressing day. Boundless misery in bruised skies. Will the weather be kind to us today?

The sun was shining on the day of my father's funeral and it made all the difference. I want nothing less for Ma today. I'm obsessed with the numbers, too. It meant so much to her that, unlike so many people in later years, people came to pay their respects to my father. I want the church to be full.

Yesterday, Martha and Felix came home from London. They are solicitous and gently caring. They are very upset, but mostly they are keeping an eye on me and Granny Rosie. My husband's oldest brother arrives, and the atmosphere is companionable. Too companionable for me. I would rather be sitting vigil, I think, like in days of old. Cold in an empty chapel, candles burning around the coffin. Contemplation and reflection, the discomfort of the pew and suffering the endless hours of the night as a mark of respect.

But today, Wednesday 14 January 2015, after the days of rain and wind, miserable weather for miserable times, the sky is clear and the clouds are new and bright.

In the garden, the grass is stiff and white with frost. The sky is shifting from a glittering starred black to blue, the sun now rising in an apricot sky. The softest tint of pink reflecting on the roof of the house next door.

Everyone is coming here, before going to the church. The same church in Felpham where my father's funeral was held. My sisters and brothers-in-law, nieces and nephews. The funeral director is ironed and smart in her black suit.

I cannot bring myself to dress, I cannot bring myself to choose.

On the morning of my father's funeral, to get rid of excess energy, I went on a long bike ride. Up to Lavant, along past the school towards West Stoke, down to the left and the long straight road next to Oldwick farm. Feeling the stretch in my thighs and calves, cycling hard, trying to out-pedal grief.

In the first few days after Ma died, I couldn't move much and I couldn't read. It was devastating that the one thing – aside from family and friends – that always gave me comfort was suddenly taken away from me. Then as Christmas gave way to New Year, I started to be able to dip in and out of books again. I couldn't bear other writers' imaginations, but books about grief. The library I'd been putting together. I couldn't concentrate much, but it seemed prudent to try to make sense of my emotions by reading about those who have walked this way before me. No book will erase the feelings of loss or the sadness, but it might help to blunt the edges. As Toni Morrison says: 'We die. That may be the meaning of life. But we do language. That may be the measure of our lives.'

And it will be words that hold me up today.

Printed on the inside of the order of service, is one of Ma's favourite Joyce Grenfell poems, 'Life Goes On':

If I should die before the rest of you,
Break not a flower nor inscribe a stone.
Nor, when I'm gone, speak in a Sunday voice,
But be the usual selves that I have known.

15

Rearranging the Chairs

MY SISTERS AND I WAIT at the lychgate, needing a little air before the service begins. Greg makes certain I'm all right. Martha and Felix put an arm around my waist, squeeze my hand, before going to take their places. The women and men from the funeral home are sombre and inexpressive. Is it my hopeful imagination that makes me think that they, too, are moved?

It is windy and cold, but a glorious day all the same.

The last few people arrive, rushing along the path throwing glancing looks of apology for being late, but I'm pleased to see them. A good turnout is what I want.

Even so, my sisters and I don't realise how good until we walk into the church itself. Walking hand in hand in hand, behind the coffin on the path, looping around, and then back to the West Door. The coffin looks so tiny, but the flowers are beautiful and our note is there. A farewell from three daughters to their much-loved mother.

A quick smoothing down of hair, then the glass doors open and the heat hits us. There's standing room only.

Standing room only.

A sideswoman whispers that they've had to send over to the church hall for more chairs and they've run out of orders of service. I'm absurdly thrilled, though it is short-lived. What wouldn't I give for Ma to see this?

Can she see this? My father would have said yes, but I don't know.

My sisters and I sit in the front pew. Behind me, Martha is crying. Felix has fixed his gaze firmly on the stained-glass window behind the altar and Granny Rosie is looking straight ahead. Greg, I know, is working hard to stay strong for everyone else. My aunt and uncle, Ma's younger brother, are here, and my cousin and her wife. My cousins on my father's side. My best friend from university is sombre in black. He's known my mother for thirty years too.

Suddenly, I know that I will struggle to get through this. When I read at my father's service I was reading as much for my mother as for him. I was caring for her. I wanted to do him justice and not make a mess of things. There was an element of duty to her and to the occasion. But this is different. There is, it seems in this fleeting moment, no one left for whom to hold everything together.

My youngest sister and another of our cousins manage their reading, slipping discreetly in and out of the pew. Then it's my turn.

It's all right to begin with. I remember my father's sage advice about public speaking – focus on the clock, if there is one, at the back of the room and try not to catch anyone's eye. At the start, my voice is steady. But when I see how many people are crying the words catch in my throat and I falter.

My children start to get to their feet, but my youngest sister is nearer. I gesture that I'm all right, but she stands next to me anyway and, looking at Greg, Martha and Felix willing me on, I manage to finish.

I say nothing more, I cannot speak the prayers, I cannot sing the hymns. The church is filled with melody, strong voices raised loud.

The priest is struggling too. He's a young man and my parents were kind to him when he first came to the parish. My sisters and I met with him to talk about what he might say and he's based his eulogy on that, but it is totally his. He includes the beautiful line – a comment by one of my oldest friends from publishing – that 'by now, Barbara will be rearranging the chairs in heaven' and everyone smiles. He adds how she had a 'busier social diary than her daughters', and everyone nods and laughs. It's a wonderful speech, heartfelt and full of personal touches – the fish and chip suppers after parish council meetings, her love of crosswords, her passion for Rafa Nadal ...

'She was a legend in the village,' the priest concludes, and though people are still dabbing their eyes, the congregation breathes a collective sigh of relief to know their feelings are shared by others. A life well lived and lived well to the very end. A Mosse cousin leads the prayers and then, it's done.

We follow the coffin out, my sisters and I. It seems to me that all is silence, as if everything is happening behind glass, so, at first, I don't hear the choir singing 'Jerusalem'. Ma's favourite hymn of all. Then, as we pass through the door and out into the afternoon, everyone in the congregation starts, little by little, to join in too and it's beautiful.

We have the committal at the gate. The priest bellowing over the wind, watching the funeral director mouthing 'ashes to ashes'. My sisters and I are holding hands, then each of us steps forward to say a final goodbye. The hearse moves off, the director walking slowly like Oliver Twist in the road in front of the cortège. People in the street bow their heads as it passes.

It's a wonderful sight, centuries old.

There's a queue to get into the church hall for the wake. Tributes and speeches, standing for hours while all sorts of people come to share their memories of Ma with us. I think again how much she would have revelled in it.

It was perfect. It was exhausting. It was the worst day ever.

When we arrive home at 3 p.m., I'm chilled to the bone. I'm not sure I'll ever feel warm again. But our kitchen is full. Martha and Felix are pouring drinks and looking after everyone. Talking and reminiscing. Stories about Ma, about my father too, happy memories.

That night, I did sleep. Eight hours, the longest sleep in months. No dreams.

Barbara Mary Mosse
15 September 1931 – 21 December 2014

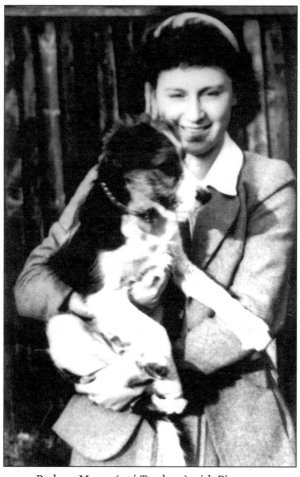

Barbara Mosse (neé Towlson) with Pip, 1949

16

Made in Dagenham

THERE ARE SO MANY OF US – musicians, nurses, singing teachers, accountants, office workers, classroom assistants, electricians, theatre directors, shop owners, cleaners, waiters, estate agents, seamstresses, managers, sound technicians, carpenters, caterers, electricians, novelists ... We are everywhere, not so much hiding as stumbling on in plain sight.

Many carers I spoke to when I was writing this book admitted how they'd often wished the constant low-level pressure wasn't there. How they felt guilty about feeling impatient, not compassionate, at yet another call for help. Guilty about the misunderstandings. How they struggled not to be resentful at needing to drop everything and rush over. Felt bad at not wanting to be in a sickroom that smelt of defeat, doing all those unpleasant and intimate tasks that have to be done over and again. That the worry about an elderly parent or parents living alone, coupled with a strong desire not to have to have them move in with them, was like a phantom ache – always there, but somehow impossible to pinpoint. That living in a world of illness and medication, symptoms and distressing setbacks, made them obsessed with their own health. When you are witnessing the worst, it's easy to believe that something bad might happen to you too. Carers often neglect their own health, but it doesn't stop the fears in the middle of the night thinking that there might be some serious illness lurking inside you.

'It's like being in sniper's alley,' is how one friend put it.

Everyone's situation is different, though almost everybody uses the word 'guilt'. Some carers have family support and split the responsibilities. Others are on their own. Cultural differences, regional differences, differences of heritage and expectation. Siblings might be estranged from one another, or have very different views on what needs to be done next. Perhaps they have a stepfather or stepmother they barely know. When a loved one dies in a care home, as opposed to a hospice or a hospital or their own bed, there is often an indecently short amount of time allocated to clear their room. Little time to think or discuss with other family members. When people are grieving, and their thoughts numbed or clouded, it's hard to make any decisions, let alone good ones.

My parents had already downsized. Even so, there seemed to be a huge number of things to be rehoused and papers to be gone through. A friend told me how she'd spent six months driving along the south coast from her house to her mother's house every week when her mother was at the end of her life. After she died, the journeys continued for another six months to meet up with her brothers to dismantle the family home they'd grown up in. For many carers, this process can be redemptive. It can restore their loved one to the person they were before the illness took hold, before confusion took hold, before their diminishing condition defined them more than the many years of life that had gone before.

It can feel disloyal to give away treasured objects, as if you're saying they don't matter. Ma had some jewellery, mostly presents from my father over nearly sixty years of marriage. She kept her necklaces, earrings and bracelets in an old-fashioned case on her dressing table. Her rings were stored on a glass ornamental tree, which fascinated all her grandchildren.

After she'd died, each of us chose something. Much of it was of its time and not to my sisters' or our children's modern tastes, and I don't wear any jewellery anyway – only a watch. All the same, we couldn't bear to let things go. It seemed a betrayal. And every moment of clearing away makes the death more real, more definite.

Some people have little to leave. Too many older people, after a lifetime of employment and paying taxes, are forced to sell their homes or possessions to pay for care, forced in the twilight of their lives to give up everything for which they've worked.

After the initial sense of freedom from living one's daily life to another person's rhythm, it's not uncommon for carers to feel purposeless when that pressure has gone. Having guiltily wished for an hour or so off, lots of us find that the days seem long. It's like being made redundant out of the blue and finding yourself standing, dazed, outside on the pavement twenty minutes after receiving your P45 with a cardboard box in your hands. The loss of a loved one might have been a release for them – from intolerable pain, or distress, or heartbreaking loss of identity, indignity as the body fails. Even so, when it's over, we still can't help but wish they were still with us. Ma had died as she had wanted, on her own terms and without decline. It didn't stop me feeling that the world was a lesser place without her.

Coping with, and preparing for, grief is a key part of being a carer of an older person. Though many are lucky to have their parents or grandparents living well into their eighties and nineties, it doesn't make the loss any less sad when it finally comes.

Ma had not needed care as such, just her family around her. Which is, of course, a different kind of care. It's about being aware, about being sensitive, about being available if and when needed. We were all grieving. All children have different relationships with their parents, however happy or equal the family, dependent on where they are in the scheme of things – oldest, middle, youngest, girl or boy, introvert or extrovert, homebody or adventurer – and the experiences they've had, both inside and outside of the family unit. My sisters and I had many shared memories of our parents, but also personal ones, unique ones belonging to us as individuals. All of this helped keep the memory of Ma, and our father too, alive.

Another common regret expressed by carers is how even the closest friendships can fade away.

During the past ten years, I gradually realised how some of the people dearest to me were around less and less. It's nobody's fault – geography and the pressures of people's working lives play their part. But it can be hard, if you have no experience of it yourself, to understand the daily requirements of being a carer. Carers often become unreliable – unreliable, that is, to anyone except the person for whom they're caring. We're no longer good friends to have: too many cancelled lunches or drinks after work that have to be postponed because something's happened and you've got to rush home. I expected people to ask how things were going, to be aware of how it might feel to be living a less flexible life, and found myself disappointed when they didn't.

Men and women who've not yet got to this stage in their lives – and may never be called upon to care – are often not very sympathetic. 'Can't someone else do it?' they think, and sometimes say. And, of course, there's often an element of truth in that. Somebody else might perfectly well be able to do it practically, but should they? If an 85-year-old man or a 90-year-old woman is frightened or confused and will be reassured by seeing you and nobody else, then you're not going to pass over the responsibility to another person, however able or competent.

Besides, you never know if this time might be the last time – the last fall, the last illness, the last time you'll be called in the middle of the night. All carers are haunted by the thought of, after everything that's happened, not being at hand when the moment comes. So, you want to be there. Every time.

Just in case.

During those first months of 2015, I existed in a fog.

I was taken aback by the depth of my grief, the absolute state of mourning. I'd expected to take it in my stride, as I had with my father, but this was utterly different. I was totally without energy, I was full of despair. Even important meetings seemed pointless. I was struggling to fall back in love with my next big fiction project, and the characters in a play I'd been working on were left languishing. They existed, but I hadn't yet given them any lines. I was working, but I was only going through the motions. Shuffling papers about the desk.

Are you still a writer if you don't write?

Then, without warning or intimation it was about to happen, there was a crack in the clouds. The gloom began to lift and, with it, the promise of better days to come. I was in London at the beginning of April. A Wednesday afternoon, on a day that was grey and dank.

I must have been going to, or coming back from, a meeting. Across Trafalgar Square, with its babel of different languages and a golden floating Yoda performing for tourists. On into the Strand. I felt disassociated from everything going on around me, as if watching it all from a great height. That vertiginous feeling when you're in the world, but not of it. The streets seemed so noisy, so pointlessly noisy. Everyone rushing. It was utterly overwhelming.

I found myself outside the Adelphi Theatre. I looked at my watch. In a matter of minutes, the midweek matinee was due to begin and an A-board on the pavement advertised there were last-minute seats available for a new musical – *Made in Dagenham* – based on the true-life story of the Ford sewing machinists strike of 1968. One of my earliest jobs in publishing had been as junior editor on Tony Benn's *Diaries*, and I remembered his entries detailing this dispute. Women fighting for their rights, for their work to be recognised as just as valuable as their male counterparts, and to be paid accordingly. Then, as now.

I bought a ticket.

Slipping through the heavy red curtains that separated the foyer from the stalls, just as the front-of-house staff were closing the doors. Whispering apologies and trying not to step on toes, I threaded my way along the half-empty row to my seat and sat, seconds before the lights went down and the band struck up.

There is nothing quite like being in a theatre in the middle of the afternoon. Everything about it is an illicit treat: the coarse white wine in a plastic cup, the programme with print too small to read, your coat draped across your knees. There's a delicious sense of transgression, of doing something naughty. Because it's the middle of a working day and you're not working, you're not doing anything for anyone else, you simply are.

The stage was a riot of colour and righteous anger, big choruses and slightly on-the-nose humour. In their company, I forgot everything for a couple hours. I didn't think of how overwhelmingly I was missing my mother, nor how my father now seemed lost to me now too. I didn't feel bereaved or guilty or lethargic. I didn't think about the series of books I wasn't writing, of the play in limbo, of the meetings I didn't want to attend.

And although it was still a drear and miserable afternoon when I came out of the theatre, I felt a little less grey. I knew something, somehow, had shifted just a little.

17

La Promenade des Anglais

I STILL COULDN'T WRITE, but in other ways I was coming back to myself. At the end of June, Greg, Granny Rosie, Martha and I went on holiday to Nice. (Felix was working, so couldn't come.)

My sisters and I grew up in the days of an annual two-week family holiday in the summer, to the New Forest or Devon or the Lake District. Because of the nature of juggling arrangements when you're a carer or have caring responsibilities, Greg and I had fallen into a pattern of never being away for very long, just a few days here or there. So it was the first time, for some years, that we could take ten days off without worrying if things were all right at home. My youngest sister was looking after the dog, so we could simply lock the front door and leave.

The days stretched out. Martha swimming; Greg sitting in the shade writing; Granny Rosie sitting on the terrace dangling her feet in the water. She needed a hand getting in and out of the pool, but trial and error resulted in a complicated trellis of plastic sun loungers and sturdier kitchen chairs, that worked. Everything can be adapted.

Other images. Rosie and me taking it slowly, arm in arm along the cobbled streets of Saint-Paul-de-Vence. She's wearing a white wide-brimmed hat in the glare of the midday sun and has her faithful walking stick for balance. My nose is sunburnt.

On Greg's birthday, we went down into Nice itself. A sedate turn up and down the Promenade des Anglais, the skateboarders and in-line skaters zigzagging in and out and around us. Music filtering up from the beach bars and restaurants.

While Rosie and Greg sat comfortably in the shade at a pavement cafe, Martha and I explored the old town and the port, the scene of so many heart-stopping boat chases and smuggling showdowns in modern-day thriller novels and films. Meandering past the elegant eighteenth-century houses above the Baie des Anges and visiting René Livieri's legendary restaurant Le Plongeoir, tribute to the famous diving boards, starkly white on their pillars of rock.

And, during those ten days, tentatively I began to write. Sitting upstairs in the rented house in the heat of the afternoon, fingers hovering over the keyboard. A play. In the cautious process of writing dialogue, I realised something else. The reason I wasn't yet ready to begin the new novel was because my last research trip, right before I'd intended to dive in, was so close to when Ma died.

The two things were tangled up together in my memory. It was a revelation. But at least my writing muscles were starting to twitch.

The Riviera was in the grips of a *canicule*, a period of excessively hot and humid weather that can sweep through that part of France at a moment's notice. The television weather forecasts were warning that those with breathing difficulties or elderly people should stay inside and reporting the soaring daily temperatures with a kind of horrified glee. Gigantic Mediterranean ants were surging out of their nests in the parched soil.

We were sensible, only going out early in the day or once the sun had lost its teeth, but Granny Rosie had a flare-up of gout all the same. A painful condition caused by hyperuricemia – a build-up of uric acid in the body – it was agonising. She's built of strong stuff, but her feet swelled horribly. It was excruciating even to have the weight of a sheet touching her leg at night.

Rosie didn't want to make a fuss, but she resented her mobility being reduced, was poleaxed by being in pain and concerned about spoiling everyone's holiday. I started to worry about how she was going to manage at the airport. I bought her some outsized Velcro sandals for her poorly feet, but there were still so many long corridors, so many steps.

We did some research. Assistance was available.

The staff at Nice airport were excellent. We got ushered through ahead of everyone else, and settled ourselves down in the airport bar to wait for our flight to be called.

We made it fun. Then, we were taken to the gate, ahead of everyone else, to be 'parked', as Rosie put it. Then the flight was delayed, but we were still left there. No more bar, no more snacks, not so much fun.

Rosie was used to pushing a wheelchair from her times looking after friends who'd needed a little extra support, but it was her first time as the passenger and she hated it. No doubt it made the journey easier and was the only sensible thing to do in the circumstances. But once we were home and the gout had cleared up, she was back on her feet with her flowery walking stick.

By October, Rosie was rehearsing with the Old Timers again, heading off to the Scrabble club at the local village hall on Tuesday afternoons and entertaining the members of the stroke-disabled club in Chichester every Thursday morning. And though, maybe, she appreciated more help getting her electric keyboard in and out of the boot of her car, she was determined not to let older age get the better of her.

I think of those fourteen months as the interim time, between being a support to my parents and becoming Rosie's extra pair of hands.

Our children were grown up, making their way in the world. My husband and I were busy with work. I'd fallen back in love with writing and was picking up the threads of my research, my planning, reacquainting myself with the characters of my next novel.

And although the first anniversary of Ma's death in

December was sad, and my sisters and I exchanged mournful text messages on the day itself, it was starting to feel like Christmas might be all right this year. We decorated a tree, we wrapped presents, we ate too much and saw friends. A photo shows us all – me, Greg, Martha, Felix and Granny Rosie, the dog lurking hopefully under the table for scraps – at the end of Christmas Day lunch, wearing lurid paper hats, the kind where the dye comes off your fingers, and with the debris of cheap cracker presents scattered between the plates.

As December draws to a close, we watch the entire box set of series eleven of *Grey's Anatomy*. I go to bed each night with the theme tune playing round and around in my head. The children go back to London. We think ahead to 2016. And when Greg, Rosie and I stay up to see in the New Year, I realise that the only hospital I've thought about for a while is this imaginary one in Seattle created by the mighty Shonda Rhimes.

18

The Colour of Patience

THERE'S A CERTAIN QUALITY of silence in the treatment centre on a Saturday afternoon. No parking wars, no queues at the barrier. The bustle of the week is gone – just those with booked appointments are there. At outpatients in the main hospital, in the COPD clinic, the cancer clinic, the day surgeries, there's a firm efficiency and comforting matter-of-factness about the ladies at reception.

There's a certain quality of light too, a milky filtered sun, a shared expectation as another healthcare professional steps out into the waiting area, all eyes rising as people listen for their name to be called. The reassuring smile when nurse and patient connect before disappearing into a featureless corridor behind the swing doors. Relief that they are in the right place, that they have not been forgotten. That they are in the system. Once the nurse and patient have disappeared, the quiet settles again, the air stills again. Waiting, again.

White is the colour of patience.

In the world of the treatment centre, time runs differently. Pushing the wheelchair through the wide revolving doors, the pattern of an office working day simply slips away. Unheard, unseen. Here, patience is what matters. The latest tenants in the rows of blue seats. There is an acceptance.

For anyone working full-time, or also caring for children, or juggling childcare and work responsibilities, this is one of the hardest parts. If you are used to a regular schedule, being more or less in charge of your own working day, this handing over of the rhythm of things is difficult. We often mistake a rigid timetable for efficiency. We fail to conceal the idea that we think our time might be, somehow, more important than the cadence of hospital procedures, than the saving of a life, than the caring for someone critically or terminally ill. Beneath this impatience, perhaps, is a deeper fear that we are diminished by being patient. We feel invisible as the person we are. Just another number in the anonymous line.

Unwittingly, our impatience reinforces what many older people feel – that they are taking up too much time. Then, they feel too much gratitude, become more anxious about their daughter or son or neighbour being kept from their 'real' life than about their illness or infirmity. For those who spend weekends driving across the country, visiting parents in their own homes or care homes often many hours away, it's even more frustrating. Should you take an hour off or two? An afternoon? A day?

Learning to be tolerant around patients is one of the first requirements for a nurse or paid carer. For us, learning to be patient around our elderly relatives is an act of kindness. To ourselves and the person for whom you are caring. It transforms the balance of things from a give-and-take to something more like equality. Two friends, family members, in it together for the long haul. Sighing, constantly checking your watch or scrolling emails on your phone (messages that, more often than not, could be left for an hour or two) – all of this makes the waiting harder. In the same way that drumming your fingers on the steering wheel and tutting does not make the traffic jam vanish, so accepting the different pattern of things, the different pace of things, is an essential part of self-care when asked to care. This, today, now, is the purpose of things. For the time being, nothing else matters. Or rather, nothing else need matter.

Any impatience a carer might feel is tenfold worse for the person who, possibly against the characteristics of a lifetime, is having to ask for help. Or even worse, not asking for it when it's so obviously needed. Not to be able to walk properly when, once, you used to run; to need help shopping when, once, the most pleasurable Saturdays were spent walking up and down the high street; not to be able to see properly, when reading was your most fulfilling pastime; not to be able to hear when conversation is one of your greatest pleasures.

We are old friends, the treatment centre and I. All glass and cathedral vaulted ceiling. The sun burns too brightly in summer and it's cold in winter when the wind's in the north-east. In the old days, I used to come here with Ma for the COPD clinic.

Now, in May 2017, I'm back here with Granny Rosie.

As a younger woman, Rosie was always on the move. A former member of a cycling club in the 1950s, happiest on a horse or swimming, a woman with a practical turn of mind and a great comfort to me after my beloved Ma died.

The spring of 2016 was blustery and wet, one of those years when the tentative blossom is torn roughly from the trees and it seems the clouds will never lift. Although Rosie was walking with a stick, she was on fighting form. Still driving, still taking our little West Highland terrier round the block for an airing. In February she was celebrated by the children's hospice for all the money she'd raised through her knitting for young people with life-limiting illnesses with a feature in the local newspaper.

For me, it was trying to catch up the time I'd lost. I was in full-steam-ahead research mode for the novel, visiting Toulouse and Carcassonne, places I knew well, but now seeing them through sixteenth-century eyes. Maps, archives, libraries, histories. Endless photographs, scribbled notes on scraps of paper.

After the many months of being crippled by grief, I was energised by my job again. I knew how lucky I was. My occupation was one I had been able to keep on the back burner. I hadn't been obliged to give it up or take all my annual holiday allowance in one go in order to support someone through a difficult time. Carers UK estimate that some 5 million carers are juggling caring responsibilities with work, but my desk was still there, my notes were waiting for when I was ready to come back to them.

In July, Granny Rosie and I went away for a couple of days.

We'd taken trips together before: once to Oberammergau to see the Passion Play, once on the Orient Express for her eightieth birthday in April 2010. 'It might be my last outing, you know,' Rosie had said as we pulled out of Victoria Station. When the official pianist on the train was taking a break, she couldn't resist slipping onto the piano stool. I suddenly realised I could hear 'It's a Long Way to Tipperary' coming over the speakers. I raced back to the Piano Bar from our cabin to find a row of gin and tonics lined up along the shining black lid and Rosie, singing her heart out, surrounded by fellow passengers asking for requests.

But Rosie was less agile now. She'd always been prone to vertigo and inner-ear problems, which affected her balance. So, rather than cope with airports or long train journeys, we went instead to the South of England County show in the New Forest.

From her earliest days with Minx, Rosie's love for riding, for ponies and horses, for gymkhanas had never waned. Carthorses, elimination trials, show jumping, dressage – for two days she watched every single event we could manage in that overcast July. I have a happy photo of her wearing her favourite printed horse shirt – a bay horse with a red-and-blue liveried rider – and clapping wildly as the heavy horses go by. We took it steady over the rough ground outside the show ring, we didn't rush and she managed.

But then, a few months after that, a moment. It wasn't the big moment, but it was the start of the next phase of things.

On an ordinary Tuesday afternoon in September, leaving our local pub after lunch, Rosie fell.

It wasn't a bad fall. Nothing was broken, she didn't hit her head. Her stick simply slipped and she stumbled, knocking into the metal planters that lined the brick steps up to the door of the pub. At the time, she was more shocked than anything. It was only when she and my husband got home that we realised she'd hurt herself. The top layer of skin on both shins had been scraped away from the bone. Her trousers, and shoes, were soaked with blood.

So many older people bruise easily and have paper-thin skin. The slightest knock, or jolt, can tear through several layers and cause a great deal of damage and pain. Often, the tiniest injury will take weeks, even months, to heal.

Rosie and I became regulars at our doctors' surgery, twice-weekly visits for nine months. By the end of it, I could recite Rosie's date of birth more readily than my own.

One stick became two. All the same, she was determined not to give in. And new novels from two of her favourite authors, Joanna Trollope and Marian Keyes, were a great help when she was laid up.

It was a tough winter. The snazzy sticks gave way to a walking frame, which she didn't take to, then a purple three-wheeler which was better. But as if that slow healing was not enough, a painful eye operation in January 2017 was followed by a diagnosis of cancer in April. Rosie had noticed things wrong 'down there'. But, truthfully, neither of us was expecting it to be anything serious.

Back to the treatment centre.

I remained in the waiting area while Rosie was being examined, wanting to give her privacy. I was talking to my son on the phone, when a low voice at my shoulder said: 'Mrs Mosse, may we have a word ...?'

It was cancer of the bladder, though caught early enough for treatment and, all being well, they were hopeful of a full recovery.

Rosie took it in her stride. The doctor's descriptions of the tumour itself – he described it was 'rather pretty, like a coral seahorse' – had us both in stitches.

Weeks of blood tests followed. The ritual of patiently sitting in more waiting rooms, listening for Rosie's name to be called, filling in forms and yet more forms. Some phlebotomists were better than others at finding a suitable vein in an old lady's arm. Rosie's hearing aid was playing up, so she maintained a running commentary on what was happening. Asking me to repeat what they were saying: 'You're on my deaf side,' she'd say, grinning at the nurse. Or when asked how she was, she'd offer

'I'm a doddering old fart' or 'I'm not what I used to be ... Nothing's what it used to be!' Everything took twice as long, but everyone thought she was hilarious. She brightened up the clinics with her good humour and quirky one-liners, and made what can be a depressing process of diagnosis and treatment into something that was ... well, it just was. As Rosie said, with a shrug: 'You've just got to get on with it.'

All the same, all the charging about was taking its toll. On me too. I was worried that she was masking any fears she might have by making light of things, but whenever I'd try to have a serious conversation about what she was feeling, she'd deflect it. 'I'm all right,' she'd say, though it had to be frightening to be having an operation at the age of eighty-seven. And it was tiring. Getting slowly in and out of the car with her three-wheeler, folding it in and out of the boot, making our way across the huge car park. Along hospital corridors that went on forever.

The operation was scheduled for May and it went well.

My brother-in-law, Rosie's oldest son, and I took her there in the morning. Twiddling our thumbs all day until we were called at dusk to fetch her back home.

That was the first time I'd been in the treatment centre at night. The orange halos from the tall streetlights glinted on the expanse of glass, the neat rows of blue regulation chairs were now perfectly aligned, ready for the morning. The ladies at reception had gone. A comfortable silence, no one rushing, like being the night watchman in a theatre after a performance when the audiences and players have returned home.

Rosie can sleep anywhere – standing up, on a bucket plastic chair in a school staffroom, on a trolley in a hospital. Once, in her twenties, she'd fallen asleep on the back of a boyfriend's motor bike going thirty miles an hour up the Old Portsmouth Road.

My brother-in-law and I got to the recovery room just before eight o'clock, to find the nurses still laughing at how Rosie, when coming round from her anaesthetic, had told the surgeon to bugger off when he'd tried to wake her up.

But any operation or medical procedure takes its toll, whatever one's age, and Rosie took a while to feel herself again and was irritated by the indignities and inconveniences of being in her ninth decade. 'I'm fed up with me,' she'd say. The combination of a ropey digestion anyway and a clash of medications had caused, in writer Paul Arnott's phrase, 'loose innards'; her balance was worse – she often felt 'swimmy'; she wore a hearing aid in her 'good ear', was deaf in the other and her eyes weren't great.

The purple three-wheeler gave way to a more robust tartan four-wheeler that had less tendency to tip.

But though it had been a bit of a tough eighteen months for her all told, Rosie was still getting about under her own steam, albeit needing a little more help. She wasn't prepared to hang up her boots just yet.

19

A Knitted Woollen Duck Pond

AT THE HEART OF THINGS, being a carer is a delicate balancing act. You don't have to take responsibility for everything. If you do, you run the danger of infantilising the person you're caring for. Just because someone's body might be letting them down, it doesn't mean their mind is fading too. Allowing choice, allowing agency, even if it means things will take longer, is a key component to caring well, caring thoughtfully.

For all of us, surely, the hope is to live and die as ourselves. Many of us perhaps, with or without a faith to guide the way, dread more the gradual decline than the inevitability of death – losing our sense of self, invisibility, the erosion of our ability to do the things that make us 'us' unaided. Most of us fear the idea of being dependent on someone else for our basic needs.

Many older people of the wartime generation, trained to soldier on, find that their bodies won't release them and are frustrated by it. My godmother, Sister Katherine, was desperate after all her long years of service, to be with God. She lived until the age of 104. Her body simply wouldn't let her go.

It is a cause for celebration that more people are living longer and living longer healthier lives. But, at the same time, we need to pay attention to the quality of that life. Living well and then having the right to die well should be seen as two sides of the same coin. The extension of life through science and technology has sometimes failed to take into account an individual's wavering desire to struggle on when their quality of life is severely impaired.

The figures for the causes of deaths in older people in the UK tell a fascinating story and highlight issues about the quality of life for older people. It's clear that better research, better and earlier diagnosis, better public health care and screening have brought about a significant change. Twenty years ago, the leading cause of death for women and men over eighty was ischemic heart disease (IHD), accounting for 18.1 per cent and 21.8 per cent of deaths registered, respectively. Ischaemia is the restriction in blood supply – and therefore oxygen supply – to tissues. Since the turn of the millennium, there's been a significant shift.

By 2018, dementia and Alzheimer's disease accounted for 12.7 per cent of all deaths registered for those over eighty for both women and men. In 2019, the Office of National Statistic (ONS) reported that dementia and Alzheimer's was the leading cause of death for women in England and

Wales (accounting for 16.1 per cent of all female deaths). Heart disease remains the most recorded cause of death for men, accounting for some 13.1 per cent of all male deaths. (It's still too early to say what the long-term impact of Covid will be on these annual mortality figures.)

There are several reasons for this shift. 'Heart health' has been a major focus of public health campaigns. Also, better understanding and improved diagnosis are likely to have caused increased reporting of dementia on death certificates. In the past, the certificate might have said 'pneumonia' – sometimes still known colloquially as 'the old person's friend' – rather than the underlying neurodegenerative condition.

For those looking after someone whose mental functions are impaired, the care burden will be additionally challenging, depending on the severity or nature of the symptoms. Trying to do your best for someone who no longer knows you, or no longer knows themselves, is impossibly hard, especially when many of those doing the caring – a wife for her husband or partner, and vice versa – are also in their eighties or even nineties. Very many elderly husbands and wives refuse to give in or allow their spouse to be cared for in a home. They've made a promise and they want to keep it. For children watching their parents struggle, this can be distressing. Is there a duty to support your mother's or father's decision, even if you can see it is doing more harm than good? Do you have the right to intervene, or persuade to another course of action? These are tough decisions to make, and more and more of us will find ourselves in this position as the overall age of the population continues to rise.

During the first national Covid-19 lockdown in the spring of 2020, when families were not allowed to visit their loved ones in care homes, the consequences for those with some form of dementia were devastating. In many places, these restrictions were not lifted even when the lockdown was over and remained in place until spring 2021. So, in the lockdowns that followed certain family members were designated as key workers in order for them to be able to provide support for severely distressed, critically fading relatives.

It was, at least, an acknowledgement that the damage done by anti-Covid measures might be worse in terms of people's emotional and mental health than the benefits of trying to protect against infection.

Rosie was frustrated by her declining mobility, but she still had an energy that would put most of us to shame.

As she moved from walking sticks to her three- then her four-wheeler 'sturdy chariot', as she called it, we were given plenty of support from the doctors' surgery about how best to adapt things in the house to make getting about easier: fewer trip hazards – rugs, trailing wires – wide spaces between pieces of furniture wherever possible for the wheels to fit through, grab rails in her bathroom and beside outside steps. We'd done all this in my parents' annexe, but now it was important to make changes in our house too.

As with my father, we had an emergency call-line system installed so that on the rare occasion Rosie was on her own in the house, should she fall, or need help, she'd be able to press the button and someone would respond straight away.

It's a brilliant system, enabling many older people to remain in their own homes for longer. However, it didn't suit Rosie and, after a few months, she gave it up. She didn't like wearing either the necklace – it kept getting caught on the door handle – or the bracelet, with its big red panic button, which was too heavy and uncomfortable on her wrist. More to the point, she couldn't hear the kindly voice that answered at the end of the line. Once, having set it off by mistake, the care team arrived to find her happily sunbathing in the garden in her bra and knickers having not heard the speaker inside the house. Rosie said it made her feel less capable, rather than providing reassurance. Since both my husband and I mostly worked from home, one of my nephews was living with us at the time and he worked shifts, there was almost always someone about or near at hand.

Back to the care company went the bracelet and necklace.

Rosie was still playing for the stroke-disabled club on Thursday mornings, but now one of us drove her car down to the church hall to unload the piano, help set it up and carry her song sheets, plugs and cushions. And though the skin on her legs had finally healed, it remained very vulnerable and she had to be careful. She gashed her arm on the sharp spike of the lavender bush. She bruised her hip on the corner of the kitchen table. Almost any slight collision might result in the immediate need for the first-aid box and bandages. By now, I was expert at applying the dressings myself. The drawer was kept filled with wound spray, disinfectant, sterile water solution and the special white surgical pads designed for fragile skin.

Despite the four-wheeler, Rosie could no longer walk long distances with much pleasure. Too many cracks in the pavement, too many high kerbs, the physical struggle of lugging the walker in and out of the car and the house.

Then in November 2017, we went up to London to see my brother-in-law's photography exhibition.

'Give me a moment,' she said, as we got down from the train.

It was a cold and slippery night at Waterloo Station, our breath billowing in white clouds on the station concourse. Rosie wouldn't have missed it for the world, but the effort of being in such a loud and noisy place took it out of her. It must have been about 150 metres from the train to the exhibition space, but it was almost too much. Though she resisted the idea of a wheelchair, not least because she was all glammed up, at the end of the evening we did ask for platform assistance to get her safely back to the carriage.

'If I give in now, I might as well give up,' she grumbled with the elderly porter, who nodded in sympathy. For five minutes, until the train came in, they happily compared ailments and medication, while I hovered in the background like a spare part.

*

If Rosie's feet were less willing, her hands certainly were not.

Having been knitting crows for the Snowdrop Trust, and Father Christmases for the children's hospice shop, she now upped her production. As December approached, she was knitting several woollen choirboys and choirgirls a day – with various coloured cassocks, to match the local churches. Each one held a hand-drawn score with the music to a different carol. They were so popular, the hospice shop had to set up a waiting list for orders. Rosie created tableaux for the window too – skiing Santas, carol singers around a lamppost, their choirmaster muffled in hat and mittens. Back and forwards we went to the wool shop. I'm hopeless with craft and art, all fingers and thumbs – I can't paint, I can't knit, I can't sew – but I became an expert in buying double knitting, four-ply, choosing the right thickness of felt for a backdrop, the right size of beads for the snowwomen's and snowmen's hats.

Rosie raised over five hundred pounds that December for children with life-limiting illnesses.

Our son wasn't going to make it home for Christmas, so my husband, daughter and I joined him on tour for a few days. My youngest sister popped in to walk the dog and my brother-in-law, Greg's elder brother, moved in to be with Rosie. When we got back, it was to find the kitchen table covered in jigsaw puzzles and crosswords. Rosie couldn't go back to the days when she taught the children how to do cartwheels in the garden. She couldn't go back to walking the dog or driving herself down to town. But she was determined to adapt and to fill her days with different things she loved doing.

'It's just how it is. No sense going on about it.'

The week before Christmas, I'm sent to buy yellow wool – Rosie was experimenting with how to knit a duck pond with chicks and ducks for Easter. And after that, perhaps she could have a go at making a maypole with ribbons and knitted children dancing for the May bank holiday.

'If I'm spared,' she adds with a wry smile ...

20

An Extra Pair of Hands

EVERY CARER KNOWS IT'S ALSO about the backup plan. Who are the family, friends, care professionals, medical support that can step in when the unexpected happens? It needn't be an emergency. It's just life. A train delayed or cancelled, a doctor's appointment running late, a meeting that goes on. These are the things that makes the difference to managing or not quite managing.

For those who have little or no support, who are caring alone or who have little financial support, every day is a matter of negotiation with social services, caring organisations, neighbours and supportive friends. It's incredibly tough.

My middle sister had caring responsibilities of her own, but my youngest sister was just round the corner and Greg's brother was always willing to drop everything to come and be with Rosie. Even so, the smallest things can accumulate and put things out of kilter.

A very close and dear friend died, unexpectedly, two days shy of his fifty-fifth birthday. He had looked after others rather than himself, but he was a ray of sunshine in everyone's life and, though I'd lost several friends of my age, it was a shock and shocked Rosie too. She felt it was wrong that she was still about, in her late eighties, whereas he was no longer with us and it made us both think about the fragility of life.

Rosie's third husband was taken very ill and it took a great deal of time and negotiation to find him a state-supported care home close enough for her to be able to visit. There were so few of her generation left now. She was worried about the situation, and guilty that I was the one having to sort things out. Pensions, utility bills, endless and complicated phone calls explaining that, no, I was no relation, but my mother-in-law was named as his next of kin and, since she was eighty-eight herself, she couldn't undertake the responsibility for his affairs.

Rosie had a few more worrying moments of her own. She knocked her hand on the door frame coming back from the hairdresser and her delicate skin needed patching up; a tumble on the cobbles in Chichester had us both sprawled down on the pavement, though we were surprised rather than hurt. Rosie hates fuss, so she was more mortified by everyone rushing to help than the possibility of having broken one of her elderly bones. Her digestion was causing her trouble, though an alteration in her daily medication seemed to make a difference. She had recovered well from her cancer operation, though walking was getting less and less secure.

After a great deal of discussion, I'd acquired a wheelchair for 'emergencies' – for journeys over cobbled streets to the shops and the supermarket, or when the weather was fine and it seemed a shame to be stuck inside. Rosie didn't really want to use it and she was aware that it would be hard to go back if she started relying on it. None of us wanted to pressurise her. Mostly, it lived in the corner of her room, shiny and red and little used. All the same, for someone who loved to be out of doors, I could see that the lack of fresh air and being out in the wider world was frustrating her. Rosie didn't want her horizons to shrink.

And having the chair meant we could go together to the Armistice Day parade at the War Memorial in Chichester, just as we had when my mother was alive. It meant we could go down to Bognor seafront and saunter along the prom. It meant we could follow Centurion Way, the old railway line, now a walking track, from Lavant to Chichester and back again. Rosie was determined the chair wouldn't become permanent – 'I don't want to lose the use of my legs' – but it gave us a measure of freedom.

Anniversaries, birthdays, children, low days and red-letter days. These are the ways we distinguish one year from the next as our lives march on. Another Christmas. Everyone was home. The tree was decorated and in its usual place. I have a photograph of Rosie on my phone reading Cathy Newman's *Bloody Brilliant Women*, a G&T at her elbow, the kitchen table covered in a thousand pieces of a fiendish jigsaw puzzle. All told, it will take a full four weeks to finish ...

When the moment happened, I wasn't there. After everything, I wasn't there when Rosie needed me.

In the spring of 2019, I went to the Netherlands on a research fellowship. Much of my new novel was to be set in sixteenth-century Amsterdam and it was an unmissable opportunity to get under the skin of the city. Visiting the archives, walking the streets where my story would be played out, learning about the history of the city, giving lectures.

I was uneasy about going and, though I was due to be away for a full month, I came home at weekends, going backwards and forwards, because it felt difficult to be away for so long. My husband and brother-in-law looked after Rosie brilliantly, but Rosie and I were pals. Girls together. Our relationship was easy and of long-standing and, because she had no daughters, I wasn't stepping on anyone's toes.

When my parents were alive, Ma had never made me feel that I was being disloyal to her by being fond of Rosie too. Putting families together, something that many carers have to wrestle with, can bring with it a complicated set of conflicting emotions, competition and stress. On top of that, sometimes an adult child is caring for her mother or father at the same time his or her partner is caring for theirs. It is challenging negotiating whose needs come first and it can often leave everyone feeling unsupported.

I enjoyed my time in Amsterdam, though I was lonely. When you have lived in and as part of a family for almost all of your life, it's startling to suddenly find yourself only responsible for yourself, subject only to your own needs and thoughts. I woke up when I wanted, ate when I was hungry, read my research notes whenever the urge took, walked all the time, wrote when I wanted to write.

It did me good, but I missed everyone. Greg was working and making sure all was well at home. Martha and Felix were working so couldn't come and visit. It was a joy when, during my last week in Amsterdam – and most of my research was done – my youngest sister and my teenage nieces came to stay. It made me think that I'd been worried for no reason at all.

It was the day before I was due home. Most of what happened I learned afterwards, in fragments of story told to me by Rosie, by my husband, by my brother-in-law.

Going to open the door to let the dog in from the garden, Rosie got her feet tangled up in her tartan walker and fell. This time, she fell properly and painfully. My nephew was there and helped her up, then rang Greg who called the doctor. Rosie insisted she didn't need to see anyone. She was only a little shaken.

But by the time I got back twenty-four hours later, things had got worse. It was clear she was deeply shocked. The undersides of both of her feet were badly bruised. She'd hurt her right elbow and her hands. Her right shoulder was painful and her shins had again taken a bashing. Most of all, it had knocked her confidence. 'I've taken against that walker,' she said and, true to her word, she never used it again.

Back to our twice-weekly visits to the surgery. Then, as summer came in, we reduced our visits down to once a week. The key issue this time was not the wounds themselves, but rather making sure that no infection slipped in. One of the bruises metamorphosed into a hideous blood blister that burst in the night. It felt like it was just one thing after the other, and Rosie took a while to come back to herself.

And though she hated the thought of it, there was now no choice but to be confined to the wheelchair full-time. 'Sodding wheels,' as she calls them. I use the word 'confined' because that's how Rosie felt it to be. She couldn't bear the idea of never walking again, but she'd lost the power in her legs. She was sleepy a lot of the time from the antibiotics and grumbled about looking 'a sketch' if she couldn't get across to her hairdresser once a week.

There were good days and bad days. But the days got longer and the sun lifted our spirits, both hers and mine, and we fell into a comfortable new way of things that suited us both. Like most women of her generation, Rosie isn't one to talk about herself. But as we sat at either end of the kitchen table, she would often suddenly remember something – a place she'd been when she was younger, a camping expedition with the children from Fordwater special school and the fun they'd had, it was like having a set of random postcards. With more time to reflect –

she no longer had any regular weekly commitments – Rosie wanted to put her past experiences in order: which month, which year, which decade even. There was no one left to ask – her twin sister had died fifteen years ago, not that they were particularly close, and all of her cousins and other relatives were gone – so we teased the timeline out together, sometimes with the help of photographs, but mostly by her working out which school she'd been teaching at when such-and-such happened.

Rosie knitting and me half-reading, talking of the trials of her marriages – always amusingly, though being on her own with three small boys can't have been easy; the day the fox got into the run and ate all the bantams; the verger's cottage which stank of the paraffin heaters; the months she lived with a stroke-disabled friend as a companion; the little house she rented one year in Devon with no running water or bathroom.

So many stories, each delivered in Rosie's deadpan way, with a shrug and a raised eyebrow.

So many tiny everyday tasks are made difficult or even impossible by being in a wheelchair.

Rosie's bedroom and bathroom had always been on the ground floor, so there were no difficulties there. But lifting the kettle to make coffee was tricky – potentially dangerous. She had little grip or strength in her wrists. Her shoulders were painful – 'too much knitting', said the osteopath, and recommended some exercises to help. She hadn't been able to go upstairs for some time and, though she didn't want anyone to do her laundry for her, there was no choice. She wanted to keep ironing, though, so we set up the ironing board at the right height for her wheelchair in the sitting room.

Like many older people with hearing aids, she found it difficult to hear on the telephone, but I could help with that. Taking messages, reordering her monthly medication, speaking to doctors. We took the footrests off the wheelchair and bought a pair of thick rubber-soled shoes – Rosie had never been one for high heels or pretty ladies' pumps anyway – so she could 'paddle about', using her feet to manoeuvre herself about.

Self-sufficient and self-reliant from her earliest days, Rosie didn't want to be, as she always put it, 'a trouble'. (Michael Crawford's *Some Mothers Do 'Ave 'Em* had always been one of her favourite television shows.) She didn't want to be cared for and wasn't used to it. But being in the wheelchair meant that she had to accept help with certain things. And though she always tried to look on the bright side, there were days when she'd say she had 'sunk below the level of positive health' or that 'I'm fed up with me'. Other days she'd say she was 'on the up'.

In December 2019, she won the Local Hero trophy at the Best of Sussex Awards in acknowledgement of the thousands of pounds she'd raised knitting for the children's hospice. I was incredibly proud of how she just carried on, doing good in the world, taking things – no pun intended – in her stride. We went to the celebration in Brighton on a blustery day – she didn't even put down her knitting as I wheeled her up to the stage to receive her trophy. Another first, as she put it. In her own way, Rosie is the epitome of Jenny Joseph's woman wearing purple clothes and a mismatched red hat in 'Warning', liberated by her age from the strictures, restrictions and traditions of life. Rosie likes having her hair done, and always matches her jumper with the right pair of trousers or a shirt, but she dresses to please herself, to be herself.

I rarely say I'm Rosie's carer and she wouldn't want me to. Even though, so far as the medical profession is concerned, it is what I am, it's not a word that tells the truth about what we are to one another. More often than not, she forgets we're a different generation and frequently introduces herself as 'Kate's daughter-in-law' or asks me where I was on VE Day or starts an anecdote about the 1950s with a sentence beginning 'Do you remember ...'

And it was Rosie, when I was talking about writing this book, who came up with the title: 'Well,' she said, 'when all's said and done, you're my extra pair of hands.'

21

The First Lockdown

IN BOOKS, IN FILMS AND THEATRE, in history lessons, we are taught that the First World War was the war that changed everything. Any event can be placed on one side or the other of those four terrible years 1914–1918 and its context is explained.

The arrival of Covid-19 will have a similar impact. Between 2020 and 2021, in every corner of the earth, the world changed and is changing still. Everything we'd taken for granted was taken away. Suddenly, we were living through 'historic' times.

February 2020 in London. I can picture myself sitting in an armchair at a low table in a coffee shop with a friend. I can't remember which one. It's late afternoon and the street lights are already on outside, glinting orange and white through the plate-glass window. When new customers come in, they bring the scent of the cold streets with them. Noses tipped red, woollen hats and gloves. I'm listening to my friend talk about what's happening in China. He says he's due to direct a theatre production in Beijing but it's looking increasingly likely the schedule will be suspended for a month or two. My memory is hazy, but I'm sure that neither of us thought it was anything more than a postponement. We didn't dream that what was happening in Wuhan would soon be happening in London. Nor that it would be the beginning of the most extraordinary ten months that most of us will ever experience.

But as spring starts to show her face, it's clear this is not local to China, but a global pandemic that will affect every country in the world.

Heeding the half-warnings and hints by the government, in March our children come home to Sussex. I have a photograph of them standing together, in the middle of the utterly empty road outside our house, still in winter coats and boots. They will be here until May. Then again, on and off, for the next ten months.

On Monday 23 March 2020, the first national lockdown begins.

There were some good things that came out of that first lockdown – less pollution, the sound of birds, cities being given back to pedestrians and the countryside to wildlife. Less rushing, less pointless consumerism, being able to spend more time with our families, the rise of the Black Lives Matter movement, more scrutiny on the American election and the possibility of change.

But the balance sheet was uneven. In the column of

deficits in the UK stand more than a hundred thousand people dead, widespread loneliness and rising mental health issues, families divided between generations, an exponential rise in domestic violence, an increase in racism, toxicity on social media, redundancy, companies going bankrupt, people dying alone and being buried without the presence of those who loved them, the economy collapsing, growing inequalities in the North/South divide in England, the chasm between those who could afford to stay home and those who had no choice but to carry on working, different rules in Wales, Scotland and Northern Ireland. The guidance changing weekly, sometimes daily.

On book tours, I used to say that people mostly never knew they were living through history. That it was only hindsight that made it so. During the pandemic, we all became aware of how we are part of history in the making every single day.

Though Martha and Felix were home, in a way things didn't feel so different.

Every carer knows how time stretches and shifts, expands, how there is a timelessness to each day, a repetition. Measuring out our lives by the daily rattle of the pill pot dispensing medication. Mealtimes. Laundry. The same conversations, though now charged by the political and social uncertainty that we cannot escape from. A paid working life is measured by hours, sometimes by minutes. Every carer knows the blurring of the hours, knows that watching the clock is a bad idea. Things take as long as they take, there is little distinction between a weekday and the weekend. Only the changes in the light and the calling of the birds mark the dawn of another day.

Now, everyone was experiencing this strange timelessness. Mornings and afternoons, the much quoted 'wine o'clock'. The fact that Monday felt the same as Tuesday as Saturday. Everything simply becomes day.

Home schooling – devastating in the third lockdown in January/February 2021 – suspensions of all non-essential medical care, shielding for those over seventy, the despair of elderly people being isolated from their families, the shifting rules and regulations as the months elide, one into the next. The erosion of public trust.

For carers, deprived of the usual support networks – the day centres, afternoon clubs, surgeries and social service providers are shut – it's impossibly hard. Having to care without backup for someone who cannot understand what is happening, with the airwaves filled with messages of the vulnerability of older people and people with learning disabilities. No one yet knows why some people get it and recover and others do not. There's a subtext that elderly people are less valued and media disinformation fans the flames.

But during the first lockdown, there's also a kind of Dunkirk spirit. A sense of community and people finally getting to know their neighbours. The weather is on our side. After the cold north winds of March, April comes in with a blowsy beauty and the temperatures rise. Walking out for an hour each day, people smile at one another and nod at strangers who are now allies in these 'strange times'.

I think it's one of the reasons that Clap for Carers took off so quickly and so powerfully. Yes, we wanted to show our respect, gratitude and appreciation. But it also became a legitimate way to glimpse those from outside of our own homes, to hear other voices, to see other faces other than those on our screens.

In our corner of Sussex, as elsewhere, it became a Thursday-night ritual and Granny Rosie, in her ninetieth year, became a media star.

At a quarter to eight on Thursday 16 April, we carried her electric piano, plugs and wires, a bloody great extension lead and an amplifier (sanitised by our gloved neighbour) and set up on the corner where three roads meet.

It's a quiet avenue of chestnut trees with their white candles proud, the first stirrings of colour on the copper beech, the sycamore with its nesting rooks. At dusk, it's a shimmering silver and green world and, in lockdown, there's no hum of traffic, only birdsong.

At 7.50, I push Granny Rosie through our garden gate and along the pavement. She is dressed up and pitch perfect and ready to play when this evening's clapping is finished. Felix helps position the wheelchair at the keyboard on the grass verge. Martha sorts out Granny's trailing wires and takes a picture. They are proud of her and she loves them helping. Greg checks the power. All over the neighbourhood we hear the clapping begin, saucepans banging, whistles, cheering, even an old football rattle, the sound of real community. The noise reverberates through every local street, large and small, gathering momentum.

Everyone has a reason for doing this. It's not abstract, an obligation, but a profound desire to acknowledge a personal debt of care. In our house, where three generations live together, the NHS is part of our daily lives. Without them, there would be no us.

Rosie's fingers hover, she turns down her hearing aid, puts her right foot on the loud pedal and, as the last echo of applause fades, she's off. It's a World War II playlist, the staples of the Old Timers: 'Wish Me Luck', 'Roll Out the Barrel', 'Pack Up Your Troubles', 'Bless 'Em All', 'Run, Rabbit, Run', 'Somewhere Over the Rainbow'.

Many of the people who live in this suburb remember these songs from their childhoods. Like Rosie who, as a fifteen-year-old, cycled from Apuldram to be there at the Market Cross in the centre of Chichester on the day peace was declared, they can remember where they were when news came that the war was over. Images in old black-and-white photographs, bunting and summer dresses, the clamorous ringing of the bells of the cathedral to mark the day.

History in the making. History as it is lived.

The sun is setting as Rosie begins her last song: 'We'll Meet Again'.

I look at all the faces and realise there are now perhaps eighty of our neighbours lining the avenues, all socially distanced, like a posed photograph. Separate in their households but, for the length of the song, together.

People start to sing, hesitantly at first, then louder as

the chorus comes around again. A mother and daughter on bicycles stop to listen. A car pulls over and a district nurse in her blue uniform gets out. A final burst of applause for her, which she acknowledges with a shy wave. An old couple dance, in an old-fashioned two-step, beneath the lime trees. Someone calls for an encore and Rosie plays 'We'll Meet Again' one more time.

Not a dry eye in the house.

The next day, my daughter posts a film on social media and things go wild. For a week, my main job becomes PR for Granny Rosie.

Radio interviews and a feature in the local newspaper. Two days later Rosie is on national television via Skype – first *The Victoria Derbyshire Show* on BBC2, then *This Morning* for ITV with Phil and Holly. We've set up her keyboard in my study so she can play live on the show, but the technology is tricky. There's a slight time lag, so I have to repeat every question so she can hear. One of her friends, now ninety-six himself, rings on the landline in the middle of the live interview to say that he's watching her on the television and she looks great! I have forgotten to unplug the phone, so it just rings and rings out in the background until the answer phone cuts in ...

Then, just before Rosie plays 'We'll Meet Again' as her finale, Holly Willoughby asks why she's doing it. Playing every single Thursday.

'Well, I saw Captain Tom,' she says, 'and I think he's marvellous. I wanted to say thank you to the NHS too.'

2 2

Wish Me Luck

IT'S JULY AND I'M IN MY STUDY, trying to write.

Granny Rosie and a 92-year-old friend from the Old Timers are in the kitchen. The entertainment troupe has wound up now: 'Most of us are dead!' she says, when asked.

But they enjoy talking about their glory days, so he comes up every fortnight once the restrictions are relaxed for a cup of tea and a gossip. They reminisce and they chuckle about the things that went wrong – the sets that collapsed, the costumes that fell to pieces, the words forgotten and the false starts.

And they sing and they sing. Verse, chorus, verse. Reprise.

I'm tempted to shut my door, but I don't want them to feel they're disturbing me and, besides, I'm not actually doing anything. I'm just sitting.

For most of this first lockdown, I've been becalmed. My writing life is relatively unaltered by confinement. I spend a lot of my time at my desk with imaginary friends. But now, as in the first six months after my mother's death, I find I can't write. I'm sleeping badly, waking most nights at three o'clock for a cup of tea and a piece of Marmite toast. Wild dreams. I've read and reread all the familiar detective stories, filling the hours before morning. And I've walked. Turning anxiety into steps registered on my phone. It is walking that has kept me sane.

I try to work out how far I've tramped since the March lockdown, without ever leaving Sussex. Probably four hundred miles across the Marshes, over the Downs, up into Kingley Vale and back, through the fields around our house. Twice, on days out, through the Suffolk reed beds and along the austere shoreline of the North Sea. I have measured out my lockdown in footsteps in the sand, across the chalky soil of Sussex, cracking twigs beneath my boots in the woods.

In the afternoons, walking with my husband to the supermarket in Chichester through deserted streets. Silence and light and footsteps somewhere out of sight. It's as if I've stepped back into my childhood in the 1960s and 70s. No shops open, the occasional car, no recorded music or the sound of the buses' engines in West Street; the spire of the cathedral always there; the Bishop's Palace Gardens, the old culvert where Greg and I sat as teenagers and watched the River Lavant run its course.

Easier times that now seem very close to me.

Our entwined lives, Rosie's and mine, have been constant during these past five months too. Martha and

Felix were here for the first lockdown, before going back to London and their partners to pick up their lives. I'd got used to having them home and they left a huge absence. My middle sister was ill with Covid and isolating with her grandsons. We missed seeing my brother-in-law and my youngest sister and her family.

But it's been a glorious summer and we've enjoyed the seasons changing before our eyes, Rosie and I. This, too, is caring. We've had time to talk about the snowdrops and crocuses, wild primroses. Every day another flower in bloom: first, the pink clematis, then the red camellia and the yellow rose, purple fuchsias and plump figs that went from green to black overnight.

Day after day we've sat in the kitchen at our usual places. In the garden beyond the double doors, scattered light falls filtered through the horse chestnut tree. In Japanese, there is a word for this phenomenon: *komoberi*. We watch the pigeons darting in and out of their nest in the yew tree. We see goldfinches and blue tits feeding on the bird table. We snoop on the unruly rooks, their nests now hidden behind a veil of green leaves as the summer progresses.

Neither of us has anywhere else to be. We take each day as it comes and, so long as I don't turn on the news and become enraged or despairing at the absolute chaos and incompetence of it all, it's been peaceful. Taking pleasure in the smallest things, as Adrienne Rich understood: 'Freedom is daily, prose-bound, routine/remembering.'

At the end of each day at around about five o'clock, an

enquiry as to whether or not the 'sun is over the yardarm' and I'll reply that 'it's over the yardarm somewhere'. A G&T and a crossword for her, a glass of white wine and a detective story for me. When Rosie gets hiccups, the only way to stop it is someone shouting 'peppermint' loudly at her – the children used to love doing this when they were little – and it works every time.

These routines of ours are comforting, in this world gone crazy. Watching *The Repair Shop* and the snooker. Her favourite is still Ronnie O'Sullivan – 'I like the naughty boys', she says. Fetching a reel of cotton from her sewing basket, locating a lost hearing aid battery or a favourite paperback book she can't find. Wheeling her to find something from her room and her reminding me to 'mind the doors', so I don't bash her into the frame. And if we are a little bored with the same stories and the same questions – 'How did you sleep?' 'What are your plans today?' 'Can you manage a little something?' – we know this is how things have to be for now, and we accept it.

Call and response, like a well-worn piece of music.

Like many older people, Rosie resents the attempts the government is making to tell her what to do. She has no time for Boris Johnson – 'Just look at the state of him!' She is indignant that old age is being equated with vulnerability and illness. 'I might be old, but there's nothing wrong with me!' My husband and I are shielding her, taking it seriously, but she has an altogether more casual attitude. 'If I get it, I get it – I've lived my life.'

I hear similar stories from other friends. That while

they are delivering shopping to their mothers and fathers, sanitising it and not venturing across the threshold, their parents are infuriated at being treated like children. Though rather grumpy about being stuck inside, Rosie is more worried about my teenage nieces and the curtailment of their freedoms than she is about her own.

In the kitchen, Rosie and her friend have moved on to 'The Lonely Goatherd' from *The Sound of Music* and are yodelling.

I shut my door.

It's August, and Granny Rosie is convinced she is on the home stretch. Not in a good way. 'I didn't think I was going to wake up this morning,' she tells me and my heart twists. It's so unlike her to be down in the dumps. She's unsentimental and perfectly matter-of-fact. 'I've had enough of me,' she says.

She might be right and I'm devastated by the thought of it though I can understand her frustration. Her shoulders are hurting all the time now and, for the past month or so, she has been on preventative antibiotics for a dangerous swelling in her legs. It's a problem common to most wheelchair users and there's little one can do except keep the legs up and try to stand and get the circulation going.

And the gout is back.

The infection and the pain and the medicine have sapped her spirits and it is demoralising for her to wake up every morning feeling a little bit worse, feeling a little bit more of her physical independence drip, dripping away. The antibiotics steal half of her day in sleep and leave her with a faint biliousness, like bilge water at the bottom of a rotting boat.

It's a Monday evening. At least, I think it is. It has the quality of a Monday in the old world. Rosie is talking about her childhood during the war. Her father was in a reserved occupation – he was a market gardener – and they lived in a tithed cottage belonging to the big house beside the church. Fresh food, exercise, a community of relatives living in striking distance. She's remembering the day they went to collect her naughty pony Minx, travelling in a trap driven too fast by her grandfather. Remembering, even eighty years later, how terrified she was that the wheels would go from under them. 'It's clearer than what happened last week,' she adds.

For years, I've tried to persuade Rosie to write her memoirs. Her memory is vivid, sharp and full of colour. She has an eye for detail and is funny, a cross between Stella Gibbons and Pam Ayres, seeing the down-to-earth humour in everything.

She doesn't do it. She loves reminiscing with me in the kitchen at the end of the day, but shies away from recording it on paper. Living above a wool shop in the parade of shops; giving birth at home and being up on her feet cooking the supper a few hours later; going to ballroom-dancing classes with her cousin in the 1940s; the uncle she and her twin sister didn't want to be left alone with; buying home-made sweets wrapped in paper through the window of an old fold-down hatch in a neighbour's house when they were six. She doesn't think anyone would be interested. All the same, I buy her one of her favourite lined pads and new pens, and resurrect the old tape recorder, thinking she might find it easier to talk her life than write it. But the stationery remains pristine in a drawer in her bedroom, the cassettes unused.

Tonight, we're talking about this book and about the nature of care before the NHS. Rosie has read something in the newspaper about the pressures on sole carers during the first lockdown and we're both in awe of the resilience and fortitude of the people interviewed.

As the light fades, Rosie starts to tell me about how her paternal grandfather was moved around in his old age. His cottage was tied to the land on which he worked. When he retired and his wife died, that was the end of the home he'd lived in for fifty-odd years. Obliged to spend a quarter of the year with each of his four children, he had nowhere to put his possessions. He was always a guest in someone else's house, often disregarded, sometimes simply forgotten.

Looking back, Rosie says she remembers she always felt sorry for him being left alone so much with no one taking any notice of him. She knew better than to say anything. 'It just was as it was.' At least when with her parents, Ern and Glad, he had a bed, not just a chair in the corner of the kitchen. On the maternal side of the family, Granny Titt (so called because she was tiny) was shunted from one relative to another too, a metal-frame bed put up in the corner of a room for the months she was there.

It's a stark reminder that when politicians mutter about family values and care at home (usually male ministers who have taken no responsibility for any kind of caring) they are inclined to paint a rosy, not always accurate, portrait of the past.

As Rosie finishes the story with a sigh and a shake of her head, I make a mental note to remember that in the days before the NHS and social services, a great many older people were at the mercy of relatives who didn't want them and only took them in on sufferance.

Despite everything, these are much better times for many.

It's Wednesday in late September, the blue hour at the end of a sunny day when the shadows lengthen on the grass and the sun begins to dip behind the trees. Granny Rosie is planning her funeral. I know there's nothing morbid in thinking ahead. It's common sense. Die we must and die we all will.

It's not a gloomy conversation – if anything it's rather jolly. But I'm aware that underneath the practical writing of lists, the looking up of readings, the printing of favourite poems, the conversation upsets me. The thought of sitting at my end of our kitchen table without seeing Rosie at her end in her wheelchair, surrounded by knitting and her terracotta bowl of essentials – a mountain of pens, emery boards, needles and threads, her pill pot, a ribbon being saved, a book of stamps – is making me desperately sad.

Though socially Church of England, Rosie is not

religious – 'when you're gone, you're gone' – so she wants a humanist funeral and a cardboard coffin. We veer off, possibly fuelled by a second glass, and wonder if a wicker or cardboard coffin is harder to carry.

Rosie can remember almost every poem she learned at school eighty years ago. One thing she definitely wants is that the final piece of music to be her singing the Gracie Fields classic 'Wish Me Luck'. We discuss how best to record it, and when. And though I feel tiny tugs at my heart – like a thread being pulled – I am smiling, because she is smiling. Her uncharacteristically low spirits of the past week or so are lifting and she's enjoying herself. I print out the words, then, accompanying herself on imaginary keys on the kitchen table, Rosie starts to sing ...

Wish me luck as you wave me goodbye
Cheerio, here I go, on my way.
Wish me luck as you wave me goodbye
Not a tear, but a cheer, make it gay.
Give me a smile I can keep all the while
In my heart while I'm away
Till we meet once again, you and I
Wish me luck as you wave me goodbye.

On her good days, Rosie is tickled by the idea of making it to a hundred like Captain Tom and getting a telegram from the Queen, though she follows almost every pronouncement with her familiar 'if I'm spared'. I want that for her too. Yes, we'll all be in bits when the time comes, but the sound of her voice reverberating around the crematorium will make everybody smile. Rosie will be so present, so utterly herself, so utterly with us as she takes her leave.

A performer to the last.

23

Rosie's Ninetieth Birthday

IT'S SATURDAY 31 OCTOBER. Halloween, though it's cancelled this year.

There are gold and white balloons, Granny Rosie's hairdresser friend has come across to 'tidy her up' before the first guests arrive, I'm putting things in the oven and bottles in the fridge.

Granny Rosie will turn ninety on Monday. Because of the rule of six, we can't have the party we'd intended to mark the occasion. So, instead, we have family and close friends coming to celebrate over three days.

Rosie didn't want a fuss, but over the last few days she's started to get excited. All of her grandchildren and, as of last week, her first great-grandchild, will be here. My sisters and their families, her nephew, her closest friend, Greg's brother and us. She's decided on a different outfit for each day – the washing machine's been busy – and her best outdoor shoes rather than her house slippers, which are better for propelling her around in her wheelchair. I'm wrestling to help her into her black patents with socks that are too thick, so instead dig out her favourite sage-green lace-ups which she's not worn for some time. Once I find the shoehorn, we're away.

Whenever people have tried to congratulate her in the build-up to the big day, Rosie batted the compliment away. 'I haven't done anything,' she says, 'I've just got older. Anyone can do it!'

But the point is, not everyone can or does do it. Her parents died in their sixties and seventies, my parents in their eighties. And though she often feels she's falling to pieces – 'nothing's what it used to be' – she is on fighting form compared to most people of her age group. There aren't many 90-year-olds who can hold their own like she can.

Every Thursday when the local newspaper arrives, Rosie turns first to the obituaries and reads the names. 'Not dead yet,' she'll say when she's been through the lot. She is only half joking. There is a courage in outliving everyone you know, but also a poignancy that yet another person who was part of your story is gone. It's why she and I talk so much. I wasn't there – we're not contemporaries, as I keep reminding her – but it helps prompt Rosie's memory. It's part of keeping that past alive. Then, the obituaries dispatched with for another week, she puts the paper aside ready to concentrate on her Thursday game of Scrabble with her friend. Sometimes she wins, but usually the game and the rattle of the tiles in the bag is punctuated with

Rosie lamenting 'I've got all vowels ...' and 'That's where I was going to go!'

The front doorbell keeps ringing. Friends and neighbours, dropping off cards and bouquets of flowers, two perfect books, a bottle of gin or two, or three, a thick blanket for her bed, a fluffy hand warmer. Rosie is the least acquisitive person I know, and is always downsizing, but everything is practical or useful and she's thrilled. There are so many cards, and though she claims to be astonished – 'I can't believe how kind everyone is being' – I can see that she is genuinely touched by this evidence of how fond people are of her.

I am touched, too, that so many of our friends have remembered and gone to so much bother. Things are tough for everyone at the moment – all the effort people have made to keep their businesses going, to keep optimistic and positive during the summer, now looks like it's been for nothing. A second national lockdown is about to be imposed, so I'm just relieved that we still could have this rolling celebration for her landmark birthday.

We all joke about her hitting a hundred. She raises her eyebrows, then adds her trademark: 'If I'm spared ...'

On the morning of her actual birthday, Monday 2 November, Rosie doesn't feel well. It's not a good day.

She's actually more worried about disappointing everyone else than how grim she's feeling, so after she's had her medication, I help her into her reclining chair so she can sleep for a while longer. Often, simply starting again – resetting, as we call it – does the trick.

Today, it does. Rosie awakes fresh and raring to go just before midday. By the time she's dressed, there's a mountain of presents waiting at her end of the kitchen table.

It's a day filled with good humour and stories. She's been telling us every year, for years, that this might be her last birthday, but this one does seem special in its own right. 'How does it feel to be ninety?' Felix asks and she considers. 'I only really feel twenty-five inside.' As she opens her presents very, very slowly – with the thrift of her generation, Rosie is determined to save every scrap of wrapping paper – she reminisces: remembering the day a horrid little boy sat behind Martha on a carousel when she was five and pulled at her plaits; the day Felix, aged six, pretended to have lost his voice so he didn't have to go to school and they played pirates all day in the garden instead; the day she locked herself out of the house, so climbed over the garden wall and broke two ribs ...

It's very noisy in the kitchen. For anyone who wears hearing aids, lots of voices together can be difficult to handle. The sound bounces, it's hard to pick out individual words and questions. After a while, Rosie turns off her hearing aid until someone offers her a restorative. 'Hold on a minute, let me switch myself on ...'

We sing 'Happy Birthday', each of us in our own key, and Rosie provides the descant. She blows out the candles and forgets to make a wish. And as I look at her shining face, surrounded by people who love her, I think of how only a couple of weeks ago she felt that her time was up. How she didn't think she'd live to see this day. In truth, how she wasn't really sure she wanted to. I think of how much I miss my parents. And of how much I love Rosie.

It's a reminder that all any of us can do – for ourselves or those we are caring for – is to take one day at a time. Enjoy the good days, muddle through the bad days, and never take anything for granted.

The next day, Rosie sleeps in late. When she wakes, she says she wishes she could do it all again.

Two days later, the second lockdown begins.

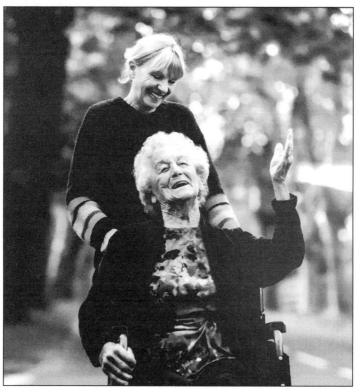

Me with Granny Rosie during #ClapForCarers, April 2020

24

Old Year, New Year

THERE'S A FROST on the ground.

During the second national lockdown and muddling tiered system, when the clocks had gone back and it was darker so much earlier, not surprisingly things felt harder than when the sun was shining and the trees were coming into leaf. We've yet to know what the real toll of these enforced periods of isolation and semi-isolation will be. For carers, many of the day-to-day issues do not change so very much: another sleepless night and cold early morning, the same negotiations about food and medication, the same medical problems, the same challenge of caring for someone at the end of their life. There is the added threat of a Brexit No Deal and with it the possibility of medical supplies being disrupted. Christmas is happening, then it's not. The emotional toll on everyone, in part because of not knowing where they stand from one day to the next, is immense. Children, parents, carers, those who are cared for. But the consequences when there is no respite care and little or no outside support, the effects on a carer's own health and mental well-being will take longer to show themselves. It bears repeating: as a society, we need to care for the carers so they can continue to care for those who cannot manage without them.

And there's hope. Not only one, but several vaccines being developed in different parts of the world – including the Pfizer, Oxford-AstraZeneca and Moderna vaccines – are looking as if they will be effective at fighting the virus. Joe Biden as President Elect of the United States has ushered in the promise of a return to politics of decency, public service and unity, though the current incumbent is inciting public disorder and refusing to accept the result. 'Up the women,' Rosie hollers, when she discovers Kamala Harris is the first ever woman, first ever woman of colour, first ever woman of South Asian descent to be the Vice President Elect, and she's thrilled to learn that Dr Jill Biden, the new FLOTUS, is a teacher and is intending to keep working. Rosie shouts it again when 90-year-old Margaret Keenan becomes the first person in the world to receive the Pfizer Covid-19 jab, then adds 'I rather fancy that spotty cardigan she's wearing ...' Martha and Felix make it home before Chichester is put into tier 4 and we have, despite everything, a lovely if quiet Christmas. Many jigsaws, the familiar old songs on the radio, too many Quality Street, paper hats and long country walks before the sun sets at 3.30 p.m.

*

As the new year of 2021 comes creeping in, things get worse before they get better. After a spike in post-Christmas Covid cases, a third national lockdown is imposed in January. This time, with no end date. Hours before children were due to begin their new term, it was announced schools would remain closed, leaving working parents with no childcare. All the strong, amazing mothers – many of them caring for older relatives too – were finally at the end of their tethers. A couple of weeks later, a Select Committee will report how the government is risking 'turning the clock back on gender equality by its failure to support caring inequalities faced by women during the pandemic'. Deaths in care homes have reached 36,000 since the previous May and residents are still being denied even the most basic physical contact with family members. In the UK, it was revealed that 2020 had the highest rate of excess deaths since the Second World War. And a new highly infectious strain of Covid was sweeping through the south-east of the country. It was the longest, the saddest, winter.

Although the newspapers were full of photographs of women and men receiving their vaccinations, Rosie, Greg and I waited for her letter, and waited, and waited. For the first time, Rosie felt vulnerable and I worried for her. 'I feel like such a drone,' she said. The cold and dark didn't help and those days seemed endless.

It was 20 January – publication day for my new novel – when the call came. I was ready in standard Zoom outfit of make-up and a smart jumper, slippers and tracksuit bottoms down below, then the phone rang. If I could get Granny Rosie to the vaccination centre in the next half an hour, then there were spaces. Greg got the car, Rosie and I battled with her duffel coat – so many toggles – and I grabbed my wellington boots. We make it to the village hall with minutes to spare. 'You *are* having a special day!' Rosie jokes, as I drag the wheelchair over the gravel in a howling wind and horizontal rain. Inside, all was calm. Several familiar faces. Rosie was wearing a shirt where the sleeves didn't roll up, so the whole thing had to come off in the church hall. 'At least it's a clean bra!' One of the nurses from our surgery administered the jab and that, somehow, felt a good sign. I took a photo of us afterwards, grinning under our masks. Above Rosie's head is the local WI noticeboard with a sign saying 'Inspiring Women'.

January gives way to February. After our initial relief at receiving the vaccine, Rosie has now 'sunk well beneath the level of positive health' and I don't seem to be able to do anything to make things better. I feel like I am letting her down. Many carers and older people have been on their own during lockdown, with no additional company. They cope with this, day in and day out. Felix is spending this lockdown at home, and this makes a world of difference. He cheers Rosie up by playing Scrabble with her and doing the crossword. But her shoulders are sore, making knitting painful, and she has a new leg injury which, despite my best efforts, gets infected. We're back to the surgery and antibiotics, which make Rosie feel even worse. Everything is such very hard work for her. Everything hurts. We've battened down the hatches, no one is coming in or out, like everyone else we have no choice but to see it through. Then on 2 February, Captain Tom dies – in hospital, from Covid, while battling pneumonia. Rosie and I raise a glass to his memory in the kitchen, but her heart isn't in it.

March arrives, wet and miserable, though there is a glimmer of light. Dates and a roadmap out of lockdown. Rosie still feels a bit discombobulated, but there's snooker on the television and a fiendish new jigsaw puzzle painting the kitchen table with riotous colour. The days pass. 'Look at this!' she roars, holding up her newspaper. Her blood is boiling at the news that people with learning disabilities are not being prioritised in the vaccine roll-out. 'As if they matter less. It's a disgrace.' I agree, though inside I realise I'm smiling. Rosie's spirits are reviving. Her zest for life is coming back. Suddenly, she's sleeping better and thinking she might manage a 'restorative', a crème caramel, a piece of fried bread even. And there are signs of spring. Daffodils on the verges and wild hyacinths, snowdrops and the first pink bloom on the clematis. Scatterings of purple crocuses.

As the weather gets warmer, we go out to take the air, a stately progress around the neighbourhood in the wheelchair to see the world coming back to life. And at the end of the afternoons, now the days are getting longer again, Rosie and I sit in companionable silence in the kitchen and watch the rooks, noisy and quarrelsome, starting to build their nests once more in the sycamore tree. We have come full circle.

Spring 2021

So, here we still live – Greg, Granny Rosie and I – with our companionship and our ghosts and our memories. In this house on the corner where three roads meet. Zora Neale Hurston wrote: 'There are years that ask questions and years that answer.' It's hard to know quite where we are. But as spring approaches, at the end of perhaps the strangest twelve months that many of us will live through, I remain ever more convinced that it is the shared stories that we tell and retell that see us through the hard times. The moments of light and fellow feeling that give us the courage to keep doing it all over again. Caring is a responsibility, it's a joy, it's tough, it carries on just the same, regardless of what's happening in the world outside. But whatever the trials of the present, we can continue to connect with one another by reminding ourselves of the things that make us 'us'. All the 'do you remember when ...?' and 'what about that day when ...?'

So, remembering driving to the Lake District with my father in 1978. I'd promised my maternal grandmother, who was dying in a Christian care home in Sussex, that I'd write a daily diary of our time there to read to her when we got home. He suggested things she'd like, memories of his own childhood.

Remembering an event at my old comprehensive school with Ma and, during a particularly serious part of the proceedings, both of us realising she was on the verge of one of her long and legendary sneezing fits. Such a delicate and tiny woman, such a tremendous ear-shattering sound. Trying to hide our laughter in our handkerchiefs and avoiding the eyes of the head teacher on the stage.

And remembering the first time I met Rosie in 1976. She was riding a moped down Church Lane, wearing a vest T-shirt and a pair of shorts, with a riding hat looped over her arm, perched on a leather horse's saddle balanced on the moped seat.

This is the most personal book I've written and is a celebration of three wonderful people – my father, my mother and my mother-in-law. I speak only for myself and don't presume to represent anyone whose circumstances might be so different from my own. I do hope, though, that anyone reading this will find an echo of some of their own emotions and common experiences.

And, of course, this is not the whole story. How could it be?

Some things are private. Thoughts or events that my father, or my mother, or Rosie would not want on the public record. Delicate things, or profoundly personal things that should be cherished only in memory.

There were many long days and even longer nights. There were disagreements and misunderstandings, all the more upsetting for being relatively rare. There were days when the relentless problems – of walking, of discomfort, of wounds that wouldn't heal, of spirits sinking lower and lower – felt too much. Too much sadness and regret for the passing of things. As T. S. Eliot's meditations on time and mortality whisper:

Teach us to care and not to care
Teach us to sit still.

There were days of anxiety and rage, impatience and guilt at being impatient. The books not written, the endless cycle of laundry, meals that no one wanted. Ambulances called in the middle of the night. Days of remorse and reproach so familiar to all carers, the sense that you are failing at everything. That I should have done more, I should have coped better.

But, when all's said and done, I'd not have had it any other way. We are who we are because of those we love, and those we allow to love us.

The Arundel Tomb about which Larkin writes so

beautifully and tenderly is in the north aisle of Chichester Cathedral. Larkin visited with his lover in 1956 and was moved to write the poem after gazing on the recumbent medieval figures with their stone hands joined in death, an earl and his countess, a little dog at their feet. Despite the ambivalence of the poem, its final line still serves as the truest epitaph: 'What will survive of us is love.'

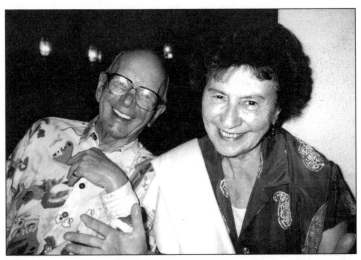

Richard and Barbara Mosse, 50th wedding anniversary, August 2004

Bibliography

This is by no means a comprehensive list, just a selection of the books I most enjoyed when researching and writing *An Extra Pair of Hands*. Some are written by paid carers – doctors, nurses, clinicians, surgeons – others are personal accounts of health and lived experiences of caring for someone. For an overview of the state of care in the UK Madeleine Bunting's exceptional *Labours of Love* is comprehensive and far-reaching. Titles are listed alphabetically by author.

The Shift: How I (lost and) found myself after 40 – and you can too by Sam Baker (Coronet, 2020)

Labours of Love: The Crisis of Care by Madeleine Bunting (Granta Books, 2020)

Dear Life: A Doctor's Story of Love, Loss and Consolation by Rachel Clarke (Little Brown, 2020)

Breathtaking: Life and Death in a Time of Contagion by Rachel Clarke (Little Brown, 2021)

Hungry by Grace Dent (Mudlark, 2020)

Life Support: Diary of an ICU Doctor at the Frontline of the Covid Crisis by Jim Down (Viking, 2021)

Intensive Care: A GP, a Community & COVID-19 by Gavin Francis (Wellcome Collection, 2021)

Being Mortal: On Illness, Medicine and What Matters in the End by Atul Gawande (Profile, 2015)

What Dementia Teaches Us About Love by Nicci Gerrard (Penguin, 2019)

Dancing with the Octopus: The Story of a True Crime by Debora Harding (Profile Books, 2020)

When Breath Becomes Air by Paul Kalanithi (Vintage, 2017)

My Year Off: Rediscovering How to Live After a Stroke by Robert McCrum (Picador, 2008)

Do No Harm: Stories of Life, Death and Brain Surgery by Henry Marsh (Weidenfeld & Nicolson, 2014)

Good Grief: Embracing Life at a Time of Death by Catherine Mayer and Anne Mayer Bird (HarperCollins, 2020)

The Fragments of my Father: A memoir of madness, love and being a carer by Sam Mills (4th Estate, 2020)

Someone I Used to Know by Wendy Mitchell (Bloomsbury, 2018)

After by Felix Mosse (film, 2020)

Who Cares? by Greg Mosse (play, 2017)

One Hundred and Fifty-Two Days by Giles Paley-Phillips (Unbound, 2020)

Duty of Care: One NHS Doctor's Story of Courage and Compassion on the Covid-19 Frontline by Dominic Pimenta (Welbeck Publishing, 2020)

The Language of Kindness: A Nurse's Story by Christie Watson (Chatto & Windus, 2018)

The Courage to Care: A Call for Compassion by Christie Watson (Chatto & Windus, 2020)

Tender: The Imperfect Art of Caring by Penny Wincer (Coronet, 2020)

Organisations

There are many national organisations offering support and advice to carers, especially those caring for people with specific life-limiting or chronic conditions. I've listed some of them below, as well as a few local organisations in Sussex mentioned in the text.

Age Concern – www.ageuk.org.uk
Alzheimer's Society – www.alzheimers.org.uk
British Lung Foundation – www.blf.org.uk
Cancer Research UK – www.cancerresearchuk.org
Carers UK – www.carersuk.org
Chestnut Tree Children's Hospice – www.chestnut-tree-house.org.uk
Diabetes UK – www.diabetes.org.uk
Hospice UK – www.hospiceuk.org

Parkinson's UK –www.parkinsons.org.uk
Sage House – www.dementia-support.org.uk
Silverline – www.thesilverline.org.uk
Snowdrop Trust – www.thesussexsnowdroptrust.com
Stroke Association – www.stroke.org.uk
St Wilfrid's Hospice – www.stwh.org

Acknowledgements

I'd like to thank my agent and friend, Mark Lucas, and everyone at the Soho Agency, especially Alice Saunders and Niamh O'Grady; huge thanks to everyone at Profile Books and Wellcome Collection, in particular Andrew Franklin, for suggesting I should write this book in the first place, my publicist Valentina Zanca, my excellent editor, Francesca Barrie, copy-editor Katherine Fry, to Ellen Johl, Natalie Ramm, Graeme Hall, Pete Dyer, Niamh Murray, Flora Willis, Penny Daniel, Claire Beaumont, Lisa Finch and the team, as well everyone who shared their own experiences of caring with me.

The reason I could be an extra pair of hands was because of the people around me. There are many friends and neighbours, but particular heartfelt thank-yous to Linda and Roger Heald, Clare Parsons, Tony Langham, Sylvia Horton, Saira Keevill, Sally Clay, Jonathan Evans,

Jill Green, Anthony Horowitz, and Kate Goodchild and Jean Graham-Jones (aka 'the girls').

Thanks to my lovely aunt and uncle Jill and Chris Towlson (and apologies for many years' worth of terrible liqueur chocolate presentation gift sets every Christmas), my nephew Rick Matthews, my cousin Anne Renshaw and cousin Phillipa Towlson-Mulbregt and her wife Kerry.

All love to my strong middle sister Caroline Matthews, who was laid low by Covid. Huge love and thanks to my fabulous youngest sister, Beth Huxley, for the 'walk-and-talk' and always keeping an eye, together with her husband Mark and their daughters Thea and Ellen, not least for epic quantities of dog walking, word grids and quizzing during lockdown. Also, to Tessa Kadler, queen of puzzles, and Ollie Halladay, for being the king of trees, trails and fire pits. Benjamin Graham is a terrific brother-in-law, always willing to drop everything and so generous with his time.

But most of all, as in all things, my love and gratitude to my beloved Greg and our wonderful children Martha and Felix. For your companionship, for your company, for your support, for the joy you bring. Thank you for caring for me.

wellcome collection

WELLCOME COLLECTION books explore health and human experience. From birth and beginnings to illness and loss, our books grapple with life's big questions through compelling writing and beautiful design. In partnership with leading independent publisher Profile Books, we champion essential voices across history, memoir, psychology, medicine and science.

WELLCOME COLLECTION is a free museum in London that aims to challenge how we all think and feel about health by connecting science, medicine, life and art. It is part of Wellcome, a global charitable foundation that supports science to solve urgent health challenges, working in more than seventy countries.

wellcomecollection.org